RENAL DIET COOKBOOK 2 IN 1

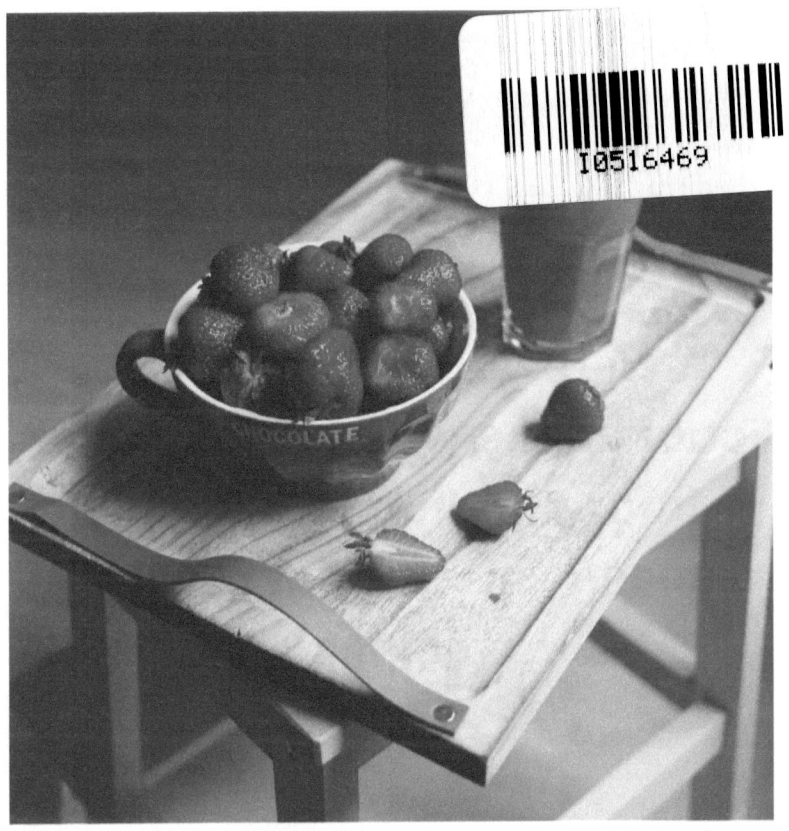

SPECIAL EDITION INCLUDING EASY TO FOLLOW AND COMPLETE RENAL DIET COOKBOOKS JUST IN ONE BOOK TO HELP YOU MANAGE KIDNEY DISEASE AND ENJOY TASTY RECIPES!

Here you will find two cookbooks with professional information about kidney disease and tastiest renal diet recipes!

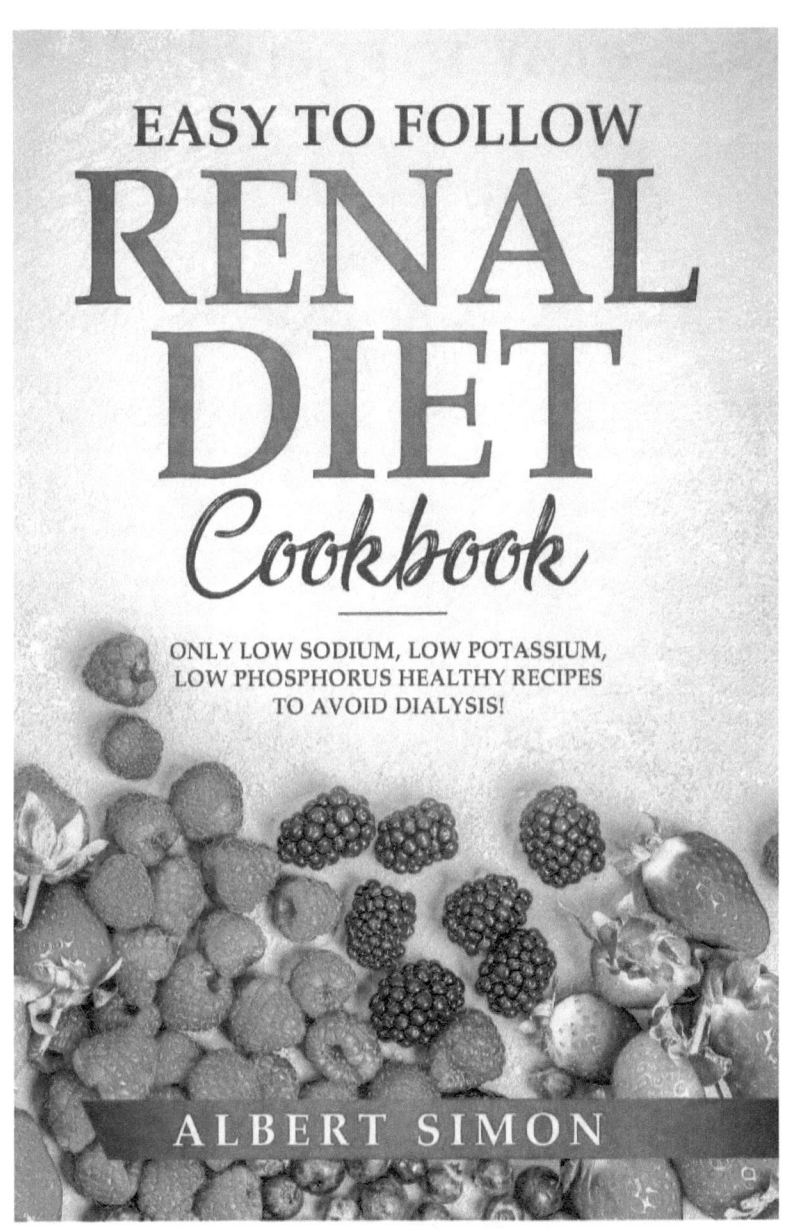

EASY TO FOLLOW
RENAL DIET
COOKBOOK

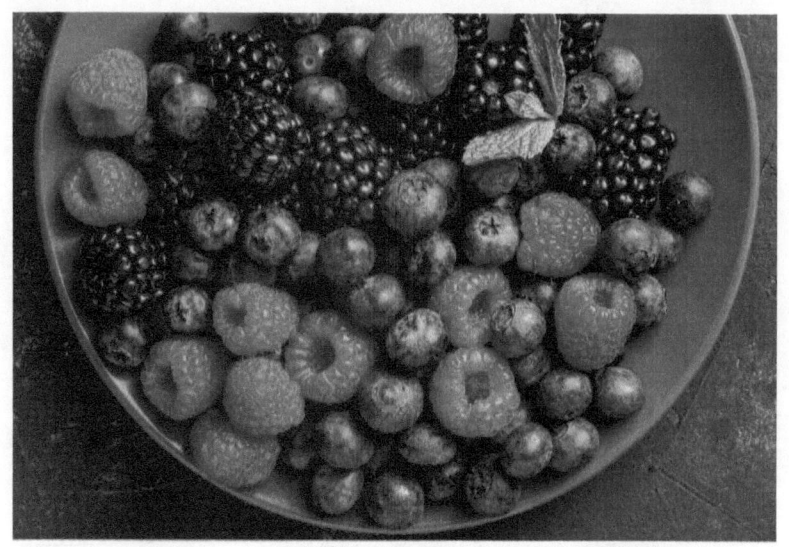

ONLY LOW SODIUM, LOW POTASSIUM, LOW PHOSPHORUS HEALTHY RECIPES TO AVOID DIALYSIS!

TABLE OF CONTENTS

Introduction 8
What is Kidney Disease? 9
What are the causes of Kidney Disease? 12
Renal Diet and its Benefits 15
What to Eat and What to Avoid in Renal Diet 26
List of Juices and Drinks for Renal Diet 30
Answers to Frequently Asked Questions 32
Best Advice to Avoid Dialysis 37
Recipes 39
    Breakfast 40
        Egg White and Broccoli Omelette 41
        Yogurt Parfait with Strawberries 43
        Mexican Scrambled Eggs in Tortilla 45
        American Blueberry Pancakes 48
        Raspberry Peach Breakfast Smoothie 51
        Fast Microwave Egg Scramble 53
        Mango Lassi Smoothie 55
        Breakfast Maple Sausage 57
        Summer Veggie Omelette 59
        Raspberry Overnight Porridge 62
    Lunch 64

Light Beef Enchiladas 65
Creamy Chicken with Cider 68
Easy and Fast Mac-n-Cheese 71
Italian Meatballs 73
Exotic Palabok 75
Vegetarian Gobi Curry 78
Marinated Shrimp and Pasta 80
Steak and Onion Sandwich 83
Zesty Crab Cakes 86
Stuffed Green Peppers 88

Dinner 91
Chicken and Noodle Soup 92
Barbeque Turkey Cups 95
Low Sodium Green Bean Casserole 97
Marinated Mushrooms in the Broiler 100
Italian Style Lamb Patties 102
Chicken with Jalapeno 104
Easy Mexican Soup 107
Seafood Casserole 109
Beef and Veggie Soup 111
Pepper Linguini Pasta 113

Desserts 115

Dessert Cocktail 116
Baked Egg Custard 118
Gumdrop Cookies 120
Pound Cake with Pineapple 123
Apple Crunch Pie 126
Easy Chocolate Pie Shell 128
Strawberry and Mint Sorbet 130
Easy Chocolate Fudge 132
High Protein Vanilla Cookies 134
Easy Pumpkin Pudding 137
Conclusion 139

Introduction

Kidney (or renal) diseases are affecting around 14% of the adult population according to international stats. In the US, approx. 661.000 Americans suffer from kidney dysfunction. Out of these patients, 468.000 proceed to dialysis treatment and the rest have one active kidney transplant.

The high numbers of diabetes and heart disease are also correlated with kidney dysfunction and sometimes one condition e.g. diabetes may lead to the other.

With so many high rates, perhaps the best course of treatment is the prevention of dialysis, which makes people depend on clinical and hospital treatments at least two times a week. Therefore, if your kidney has already shown some signs of dysfunction, you can prevent dialysis through diet, something that we are going to discuss in this book.

What is Kidney Disease?

A kidney disease diagnosis implies that the kidneys are either dysfunctional, under-functioning, or damaged and cannot filter out toxins and metabolic waste on their own. Our systems need our kidneys for a waste filtering process. However, when kidney damage occurs, the system is piled up with damaging waste that it cannot expel through other means. As a result, inflammatory responses emerge and you have a much higher chance of developing chronic and serious health disorders like diabetes or heart failure, which can even be fatal in extreme cases.

There are two main types of kidney disease, based on their cause and time duration:

- **Sudden and unexpected kidney damage/acute kidney injury (AKI)** as a result of an accident or surgery side effects, which usually lasts for a short period.

- **Chronic and progressive kidney dysfunction (CKD).** As its name suggests, this is a chronic condition with multiple progressive stages that lead ultimately to permanent kidney damage. There are approx. 5 stages of the disorder and during the last and final stage, the patient will need dialysis or a kidney transplant to survive. This final stage is also known in the medical glossary as End-Stage-Renal Disease (ESRD).

During all kidney dysfunction stages, there are higher than normal amounts of a certain protein called *Arbutin* in the urine, which can be confirmed by urine tests for diagnosing renal disease. This condition is known scientifically as *Proteinuria*. Doctors may also perform blood tests and/or image screening tests to pinpoint a problem with the kidneys and come up with a diagnosis.

What are the causes of Kidney Disease?

Chronic kidney disease is often the result of other chronic health conditions. Diabetes, according to medical stats, is the leading cause of kidney dysfunction and ultimately ESRD. Other common causes include:

- Elevated blood pressure
- Autoimmune problems and disorders such as Lupus, celiac disease, and IgA nephropathy.
- Urinary tract problems and infections
- Nephrotic syndrome (a condition that results in abnormal levels of protein in the urine while the actual protein levels in the blood are low).

In some cases, kidneys may cease to function unexpectedly for a very brief period that is usually a couple of days. This is the result of an accident or sudden body failures like:

- Heart attack
- Drug and substance abuse
- Insufficient blood flow to the kidneys
- Urinary tract infections

In this case, the kidney damage is only temporary and your kidneys will switch back to their normal function after just a couple of days, especially if you don't have any other chronic health problems that will affect their recovery.

The problem is, kidney damage at first doesn't show any symptoms that you can notice on your own and it's no wonder why many people call it a "silent disease". The symptoms usually are more noticeable during the last stages of the disease and include:

- Fatigue for no reason
- A feeling of coldness and numbness
- Breath problems e.g. shortness of breath
- Weakness and tiredness
- Dizziness, nausea

- Cognitive problems e.g. trouble concentrating and thinking clearly
- Swelling of hands and feet
- Swelling and puffiness or redness in the face
- Change in taste sensations/food appears to have a metal taste
- Ammonia/bad breath
- Tendency to vomit
- Itchiness
- Bubbly and burning urine
- Red, brown, or purple urine
- Intense pressure needed to urinate

Many of the above symptoms though can be a sign of other health conditions e.g. inflammatory bowel disease and so if you have any of the above mentioned, you have to consult with a doctor for a proper diagnosis and before the condition gets worse.

Renal Diet and its Benefits

If you have been diagnosed with kidney dysfunction, a proper diet is necessary for controlling the amount of toxic waste in the bloodstream. When toxic waste piles up in the system along with increased fluid, chronic inflammation occurs and we have a much higher chance of developing cardiovascular, bone, metabolic, or other health issues.

Since your kidneys can't fully get rid of the waste on their own, which comes from food and drinks, probably the only natural way to help our system is through this diet.

A renal diet is especially useful during the first stages of kidney dysfunction and leads to the following benefits:

- Prevents excess fluid and waste build-up
- Prevents the progression of renal dysfunction stages

- Decreases the likelihood of developing other chronic health problems e.g. heart disorders
- Has a mild antioxidant function in the body, which keeps inflammation and inflammatory responses under control.

The above-mentioned benefits are noticeable once the patient follows the diet for at least a month and then continuing it for longer periods, to avoid the stage where dialysis is needed. The strictness of the diet depends on the current stage of renal/kidney disease, if, for example, you are in the 3rd or 4th stage, you should follow a more strict diet and be attentive to the food, which is allowed or prohibited.

These exact foods and nutrients that you should take when following a renal diet, will be given to you in the following sections, so keep on reading.

Explanation of key diet words

The following nutrients play a major role in a renal diet as some have the ability to improve the condition while others can make it worse. Essentially, a renal diet is based on low consumption of certain nutrients like potassium and phosphorus simply because it promotes fluid buildup within the system of a kidney patient. Here is a brief explanation of the function of each nutrient and its role in a renal diet:

Potassium.

Potassium is a mineral that naturally occurs in certain foods and plays a role in regulating heart rhythm and muscle movement. It is also needed for keeping fluid and electrolyte balance at normal levels. Our kidneys keep only the right levels of potassium in our system, and when it is excess, they expel it via the urine.

The problem is, once kidneys can't function properly, all this excess potassium can't be expelled out and spikes up, causing symptoms like muscle and bone weakness, abnormal heartbeat, and heart failure in extreme cases.

Thus, a diet low in potassium is recommended to prevent buildup and avoid such negative side effects.

Sodium.

Sodium is a trace mineral that is found in most foods that we eat today and it is the key component of salt, which is actually a sodium compound mixed with chloride. Most food that we consume and specially processed food is highly loaded with salt, however, we may be eating sodium in other forms too e.g. fish. The key role of sodium is to regulate blood pressure, help regulate nerve function, and maintain the balance of acids in the blood. However, when sodium is excessively high and the kidneys can expel it, it can lead to the following symptoms: an elevated feeling of thirst, swelling of hands, feet, and face, elevated blood pressure, and problems with breathing. This is why it is suggested to keep sodium intake low.

Phosphorus.

Phosphorus is an essential mineral that is responsible for the development and regeneration of our bones. Phosphorus also plays a key role in the growth of connective tissue e.g. muscles and the regulation of muscle motions. When the food we take contains phosphorus, it gets absorbed by the intestines and then gets deposited in our bones.

However, when kidneys are damaged or dysfunctional, the excess phosphorus can't be expelled through our systems and causes problems such as: extracting calcium out of the bones/making them weaker, and leading to excess calcium in the bloodstream which interferes with blood vessels, heart, eye, and lung function.

Protein.

Protein is a nutritional compound that consists of amino acids, which play a key role in various system functions like cell communication, oxygen supply, and cellular metabolism. They are also a part of a healthy immune system.

Normally, protein is not an issue for our kidneys. When protein is metabolized, waste by-products are also created and are filtered through the kidneys. This waste along with extrarenal proteins after will be expelled through urine.

However, when kidneys are unable to filter out excess protein, it gets accumulated in the blood and cause problems.

This doesn't mean that renal disease patients should avoid protein totally as it is still necessary for some metabolic functions, as long as it's taken in moderate amounts and based on the stage of renal disease.

Carbs.

Carbs act as a key source of fuel for our bodies. The consumption of carbs is turned into glucose in our system, which is a primary source of energy.

Carbs are ok to be eaten in moderation by kidney patients and the daily recommended allowance is up to 150 grams/day. However, patients that also suffer from Diabetes (besides renal disease) should control their carb consumption to avoid any sudden spikes in their blood glucose.

Fats.

Being in balanced amounts, fats in our bodies act as an energy source, aid in the release of hormones, and help regulate blood pressure. They also carry some vitamins that are fat-soluble such as A, D, E, and K, which are also very important for our systems. Not all fats are created equal though, some are good for our health and some are bad. Bad fats are saturated and trans fats that usually exist in processed meat, dairy, and other products. They are also found in margarine and vegetable fat shortenings.

Fats, in general, don't pose a risk for renal disease patients, however, it is suggested to limit the consumption of saturated and trans fats to avoid any cardiovascular problems e.g. elevated blood pressure and clogging of the arteries.

Dietary fiber.

Dietary fiber is a compound that can't be digested on its own by enzymes and acids in our stomach and intestines but is needed for the system to aid in the digestion of our food and encourage bowel movements. They generally promote bowel regularity and decrease the likelihood of developing constipation inside the colon. Dietary fiber is typically found in fruits, vegetables, seeds, and whole grains.

In patients with renal disease, dietary fiber is ok up to 28 grams/day as long as these plant foods don't contain high amounts of phosphorus or potassium.

Vitamins.

According to medical and dietary guidelines, our bodies need close to 13 vitamins to functions. Vitamins play a key role in metabolic functions and the normal functioning of our cardiovascular, digestive, nervous system and immune systems. The adoption of a nutritionally dense and balanced diet is necessary for getting all the vitamins our system needs. However, due to some diet restrictions e.g. sodium, many renal patients need water-soluble vitamins like B-complex (B1, B2, B6, B12, folic acid, biotin) and small amounts of Vitamin C.

Minerals.

Minerals are needed for our system to maintain healthy connective tissue e.g. bones, muscles, and skin, and facilitate the normal function of our hearts and central nervous systems.

Our kidneys typically expel any excess amount of minerals through our urine as some can lead to health symptoms e.g. muscle spasms when their levels are abnormally high.

However, as it was mentioned earlier, some minerals like potassium and phosphorus cannot be expelled by our kidneys when in excess and so their intake through diet should be limited.

Other trace minerals are perfectly fine when following a renal diet: iron, copper, zinc, and selenium. A lack of these can lead to increased oxidative stress and thus, it is important to take sufficient amounts through diet or supplementation.

Fluids.

Fluids are necessary for the proper hydration of our systems, in fact, lack of fluids can lead to dehydration and death in extreme cases.

However, in patients with renal dysfunction, fluids can quickly build-up to the point of placing pressure on vital organs like the lungs and heart and becoming dangerous. This is the reason why many physicians advise their kidney patients to limit the consumption of fluids, especially during the last stages of the disorder.

What to Eat and What to Avoid in Renal Diet

As specified above, some nutrients should be limited in the renal diet e.g. phosphorus, potassium, and thus any foods that contain high amounts of these should be taken only in low amounts and not on a daily basis. The foods that should be limited are:

- Bananas
- Avocadoes
- Beetroots
- Dried beans
- Dried fruit
- Mangos
- Melons
- Molasses
- Nuts and seeds
- Oranges
- Parsnips

- Spinach
- Potatoes
- Fish
- Low-fat yogurt

Be attentive! Following foods have a high amount of sodium and their consumption should be limited:

- Salty snacks e.g. pretzels, potato chips, packed popcorn, etc.
- Savory pies e.g. cheese pies, sausage rolls, and Greek spinach pies
- Processed meats e.g. luncheon meat, salami, sausages
- Pickled foods in salt brine
- Condiments e.g. ketchup, mustard, and mayo
- Soy sauce
- Canned soups and sauces

Now, here are the top foods you can consume without any (strict) restrictions, as they are naturally low in potassium, phosphorus, and sodium:

- Cabbage
- Cucumber
- Broccoli
- Cauliflower
- Brussels sprouts
- Onions
- Garlic
- Apples
- Berries (blueberries, cranberries, berries, strawberries)
- Cherries
- Red grapes
- Egg whites
- Wild-caught fish
- Olive oil
- Bulgur wheat
- Oatmeal
- Skinless chicken and turkey
- Arugula

- Macadamia Nuts
- Radishes
- Shiitake mushrooms
- Pineapple
- Grapefruits
- Kale
- Ginger
- All spices and herbs

Red meat and dairy can also be consumed in moderation but they should not be combined with high phosphorus, potassium, or sodium foods as they contain moderate amounts of these alone.

List of Juices and Drinks for Renal Diet

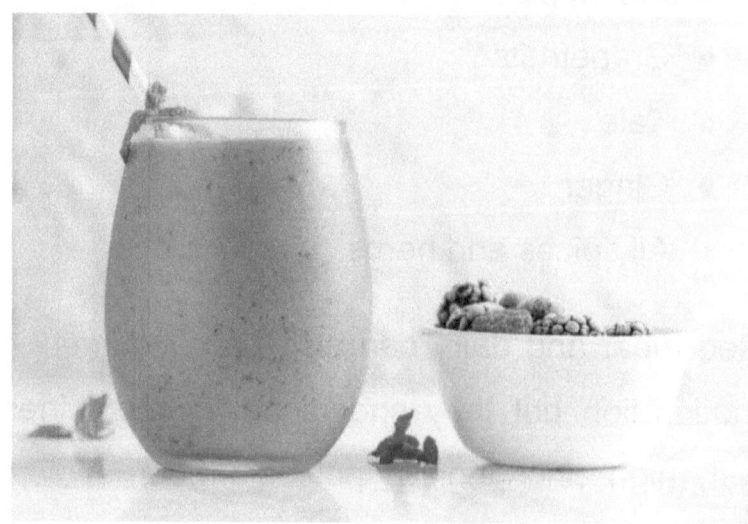

If you wish sufficiently hydrate yourself without increasing your sodium, phosphorus, or potassium intake, there are a few drinks and juices you can drink regularly:

- Freshly made apple juice
- Berry juices
- Red wine (up to two glasses a day)
- Grape juice
- Filtered drinking water

- Pineapple juice
- Cucumber juice
- Lemon juice diluted
- Most unsweetened herbal tea e.g. green tea, mint, ginger, cinnamon, etc.
- Coffee (in moderation)

During the late stages of renal dysfunction and particularly from stage 3, as usual, physicians recommend the limitation of fluids up to 1500 mg/day (which is equal to 5-6 glasses of liquids per day). However, this is something that you'd better discuss with your doctor as adjusting the amount yourself may lead to fluid imbalance.

Answers to Frequently Asked Questions

When you are diagnosed with renal disease, it is perfectly natural and common to have some questions in regards to kidney function and renal diet. Here are the most common questions and their answers in brief:

Q: How much protein should I take daily?
A: The exact amount of protein you should take per day depends on your existing body weight, stage of renal disease, and general health status. This is something that you can figure out with your doctor or renal dietitian. However, in most cases, doctors recommend the approx. 1.1-1.3 grams of protein per kg of body weight daily. For example, if you weigh 143Pounds/65Kg, you can eat up to 84 grams of protein per day without any problems.

Q: Do I need to take extra vitamins and supplements?

A: Due to the fact that a lot of nutrient-dense foods should be avoided in a renal diet because of their high potassium or phosphorus content, it is generally suggested to take vitamins that are water-soluble and namely B-complex vitamins and vitamin C in smaller doses. However, excess supplementation may lead to side effects like stomach irritation, gas and constipation so make sure you do not exceed the daily-recommended dose on the package.

Q: Are alcoholic beverages ok to drink in a renal diet?

A: Drinks that contain lower amounts of alcohol than others e.g. wine and beer are fine to drink on a semi-regular basis e.g. 2-3 times a week. However, heavy alcoholic drinks like vodka, rum, tequila, gin, and whiskey should be limited to 2-3 times a month, as frequent consumption will place kidneys and other vital organs under stress.

Q: How can I figure out if a packed food product or recipe is low in potassium?

A: When you are checking a product label or new recipe but don't know if it's actually low in potassium or not, here is a basic guideline of levels per serving:

Very low potassium levels	up to 35 mg/serving
Low potassium levels	up to 150 mg/serving
Moderate potassium levels	Between 150-250 mg/serving
High potassium levels	250-500 mg/serving
Very high potassium levels	500mg+/serving

If you are checking a recipe, make sure that you calculate the total levels of all ingredients to determine the amount of potassium. In this book, we made it easier for you by including recipes that are low or moderate in potassium and display the actual potassium level per serving.

Q: Do I have to limit my fluids after being diagnosed?

A: A limitation of fluids is generally recommended during the last stages of kidney damage and it would be better to discuss with your doctor. If you go opposite and only drink 500ml of fluids or less per day, you risk dehydrating yourself and cause other problems.

Q: Are artificial sweeteners OK in the renal diet?

A: Artificial sweeteners that are low in carbs are generally fine to the consumer within the renal diet except for aspartame which is linked to many health problems, sweeteners like stevia, sucralose, and xylitol are perfectly fine when consumed moderately on a regular basis.

Q: Can I follow this diet if I have a kidney transplant?

A: Although this diet is designed to help patients of nearly all stages of kidney damage, once you have a kidney transplant surgery, you may follow afterward a similar diet but your protein requirements will be higher, as your body will need extra protein to heal damaged tissue. In addition, maybe you will need to eat higher amounts of calcium to avoid any depletion because of steroid medications. The exact diet and portions are something that you will discuss with your doctor or renal dietician post-surgery.

Best Advice to Avoid Dialysis

As specified, if you are currently in the first stages of renal damage, you can prevent dialysis mainly through diet, but other general lifestyle factors will help. As a rule of thumb, you need to follow a lifestyle that keeps your body weight under control and makes you feel healthy. Here are some tips:

Exercise regularly. It is important to be physically active to keep your heart and breathing system healthy, as renal damage can also affect their functions as well. Most doctors recommend exercising 2-3 times a week and performing mild exercises to keep yourself active but not too tired or exhausted. Three hours in total of mild exercise per week is perfectly fine for this purpose.

Monitor your blood sugar levels. Blood sugar levels and diabetes are often a side effect or even a contributing factor to renal damage. Even if you don't have currently diabetes, it is still important to monitor your blood sugar levels as they can place you at risk of developing renal disease further. Check them at least once a month and if you are in pre-diabetes or full set diabetes status, make sure that you take all the medicines that your doctor prescribes for your case.

Keep your immune system balanced. When our immune systems are underactive or overactive, many types of diseases can occur as a result of the body's inability to fight them properly. In the case of renal disease, some autoimmune conditions like Lupus are negatively associated with the progression of the disease. In this case, your doctor may prescribe steroids to keep your immune system from getting over-triggered and attacking vital organs e.g. kidneys.

Recipes

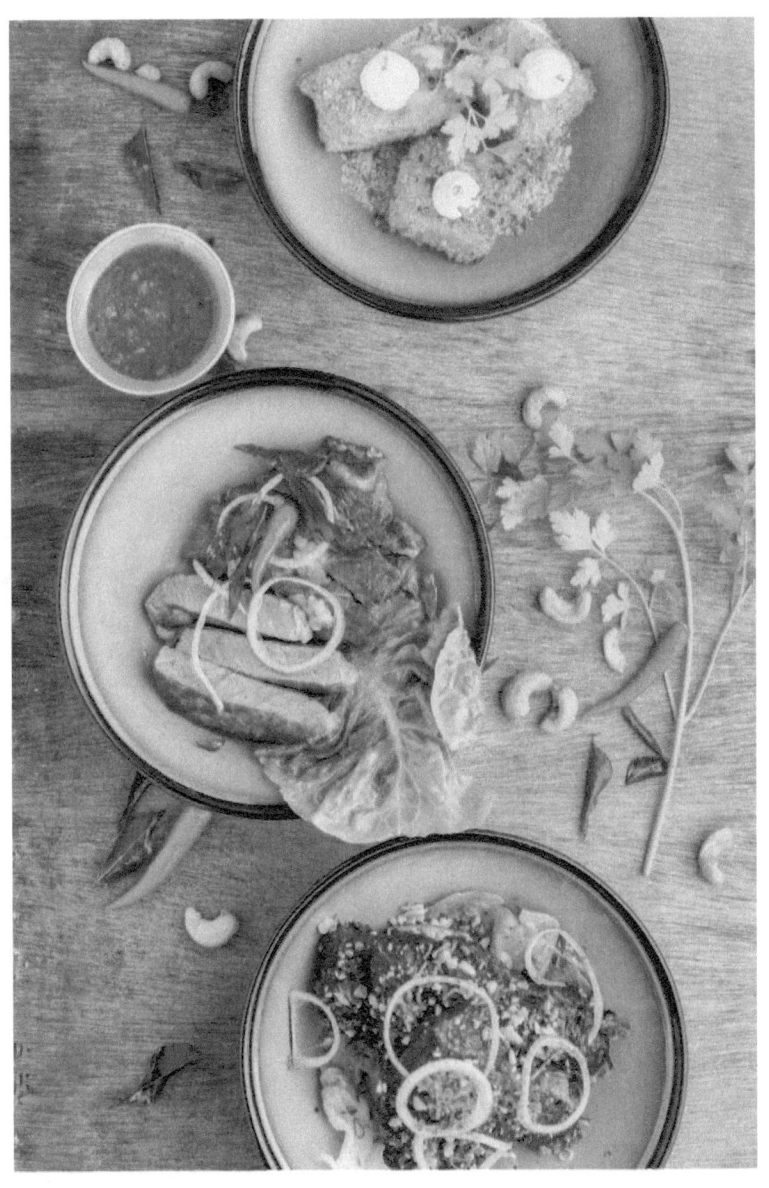

Breakfast

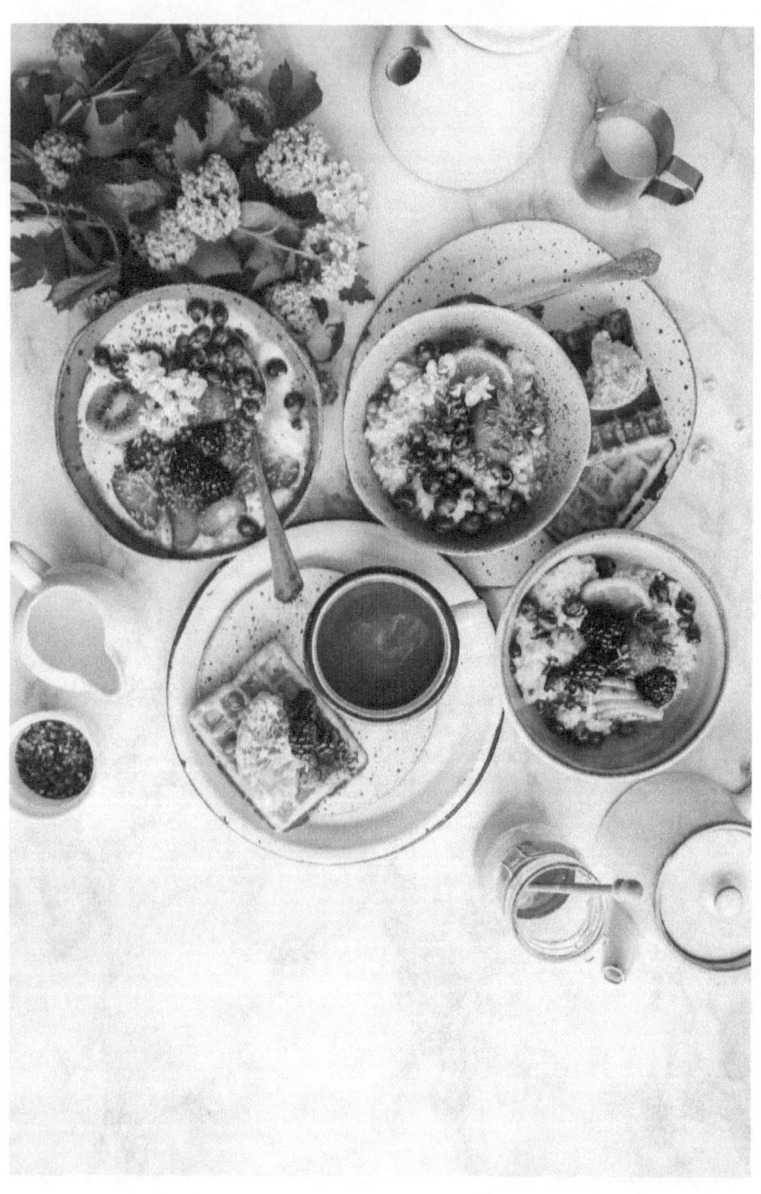

Egg White and Broccoli Omelette

COOKING TIME: 4 MINUTES

DESCRIPTION

A light, tasty, and incredibly fluffy omelet with egg whites, broccoli, and a bit of extra cheese on top that is perfect for brunch or breakfast. Ready in just 5 minutes.

INGREDIENTS FOR 2 SERVINGS

- 4 egg whites
- 1/3 cup of boiled broccoli
- ½ tsp of Dill
- 1 tbsp of parmesan cheese, grated
- Salt/Pepper

METHOD

1. In a small bowl, beat together the egg whites until stiff and white.
2. Add the dill, the broccoli, and the parmesan cheese, and incorporate

everything with a spatula (do not over whisk).
3. Spray the pan with a bit of cooking spray and pour the egg and broccoli mixture. Cook around 1-2 minutes on each side.
4. Turn the omelet in half and optionally garnish with just a little bit of cheese on top.

NUTRITIONAL INFORMATION (Per Serving)

- Calories: 56.82 kcal
- Carbohydrate: 2.7 g
- Protein: 10.57 g
- Sodium: 271.9 mg
- Potassium: 168.74 mg
- Phosphorus: 50.8 mg
- Dietary Fiber: 0.79 g
- Fat: 1.65 g
- Sugar: 1.46 g

Yogurt Parfait with Strawberries

COOKING TIME: 1 MINUTE

DESCRIPTION

Do you need something fresh and sweet for breakfast? If yes, you can try this yogurt parfait with strawberries that will be ready in a minute and it is loaded with vanilla powder for extra protein.

INGREDIENTS FOR 2 SERVINGS

- ½ cup of soy yogurt (plain)
- 1 scoop of vanilla flavored protein
- 5 fresh strawberries, sliced
- 1 tbsp of agave syrup

METHOD

1. In a bowl, slowly whisk the protein powder with the yogurt.

2. Add the strawberry slices and the agave syrup on top.
3. Serve.

NUTRITIONAL INFORMATION (Per Serving)

- Calories: 153.25 kcal
- Carbohydrate: 23.5 g
- Protein: 12.67 g
- Sodium: 93.32 mg
- Potassium: 85.9 mg
- Phosphorus: 62.75 mg
- Dietary Fiber: 1.43 g
- Fat: 1.17 g
- Sugar: 6.9 g

Mexican Scrambled Eggs in Tortilla

COOKING TIME: 2 MINUTES

DESCRIPTION

A hearty egg recipe inspired by the true Mexican flavors of chilies and cumin, which is easy to make and has an incredible taste. Perfect for a brunch for two.

INGREDIENTS FOR 2 SERVINGS

- 2 medium corn tortillas
- 4 egg whites
- 1 tsp of cumin
- 3 tsp of green chilies, diced
- ½ tsp of hot pepper sauce
- 2 tbsp of salsa
- ½ tsp salt

METHOD

1. Spray some cooking spray on a medium skillet and heat for a few seconds.
2. Whisk the eggs with green chilies, hot sauce, and cumin.
3. Add the eggs into the pan, and whisk with a spatula to scrumble. Add the salt.
4. Cook until fluffy and done (1-2 minutes) over low heat.
5. Open the tortillas and spread 1 tbsp of salsa on each.
6. Distribute the egg mixture onto the tortillas and wrap gently to make a burrito.
7. Serve warm.

NUTRITIONAL INFORMATION (Per Serving)

- Calories: 44.1 kcal
- Carbohydrate: 2.23 g
- Protein: 7.69 g
- Sodium: 854 mg
- Potassium: 189 mg
- Phosphorus: 22 mg

- Dietary Fiber: 0.5 g
- Fat: 0.39 g
- Sugar: 1.4 g

American Blueberry Pancakes

COOKING TIME: 10 MINUTES

DESCRIPTION

Everyone loves good old-pancakes that remind us of those that our grandmas used to make. The addition of blueberries here adds a nice tangy twist while keeping phosphorus and potassium levels low.

INGREDIENTS FOR 6 SERVINGS

- 1 ½ cups of all-purpose flour, sifted
- 1 cup of buttermilk
- 3 tbsp of sugar
- 2 tbsp of unsalted butter, melted
- 2 tsp of baking powder
- 2 eggs, beaten
- 1 cup of canned blueberries, rinsed

METHOD

1. Combine the flour, baking powder, and sugar in a bowl.
2. Make a hole in the center and slowly add the rest of the ingredients.
3. Begin to stir gently from the sides to the center with a spatula, until you get a smooth and creamy batter.
4. Spray a small pan with cooking spray and place over medium heat.
5. Take one measuring cup and fill 1/3rd of its capacity with the batter to make each pancake.
6. Use a spoon to pour the pancake batter and let cook until golden brown. Flip once to cook the other side.
7. Serve warm with optional agave syrup.

NUTRITIONAL INFORMATION (Per Serving)

- Calories: 251.69 kcal
- Carbohydrate: 41.68 g
- Protein: 7.2 g
- Sodium: 186.68 mg

- Potassium: 142.87 mg
- Phosphorus: 255.39 mg
- Dietary Fiber: 1.9 g
- Fat: 6.47 g
- Sugar: 5.53 g

Raspberry Peach Breakfast Smoothie

COOKING TIME: 1 MINUTE

DESCRIPTION

A bright, rich, and zesty smoothie for kick-starting your day with energy and nutrients that will keep you until lunch.

INGREDIENTS FOR 2 SERVINGS

- 1/3 cup of raspberries, (it can be frozen)
- 1/2 peach, skin, and pit removed
- 1 tbsp of honey
- 1 cup of coconut water

METHOD

1. Combine all the ingredients in a blender until smooth.
2. Pour and serve chilled in a tall glass or mason jar.

NUTRITIONAL INFORMATION (Per Serving)

- Calories: 86.3 kcal
- Carbohydrate: 20.6 g
- Protein: 1.4 g
- Sodium: 3 mg
- Potassium: 109 mg
- Phosphorus: 36.08 mg
- Dietary Fiber: 2.6 g
- Fat: 0.31 g
- Sugar: 16.8 g

Fast Microwave Egg Scramble

COOKING TIME: 1-2 MINUTES

DESCRIPTION

Do you need your eggs extra fast without getting stuff dirty? You can try this 1 ½ minute scramble microwave recipe that is low in phosphorus and moderate to low in potassium levels as well.

INGREDIENTS FOR 1 SERVING

- 1 large egg
- 2 large egg whites
- 2 tbsp of milk
- Kosher pepper, ground

METHOD

1. Spray a coffee cup with a bit of cooking spray.

2. Whisk all the ingredients together and place them into the coffee cup.
3. Place the cup with the eggs into the microwave and set to cook for approx. 45 seconds. Take out and stir.
4. Return to the microwave and cook for another 30 seconds.
5. Serve.

NUTRITIONAL INFORMATION (Per Serving)

- Calories: 128.6 kcal
- Carbohydrate: 2.47 g
- Protein: 12.96 g
- Sodium: 286.36 mg
- Potassium: 185.28 mg
- Phosphorus: 122.22 mg
- Dietary Fiber: 0 g
- Fat: 5.96 g
- Sugar: 2 g

Mango Lassi Smoothie

COOKING TIME: 1 MINUTE

DESCRIPTION

This smoothie recipe stands out from the rest in its rich exotic aroma and zesty flavor, thanks to a smart combination of mango and spices like cinnamon and cardamom. Great for breakfast or post or pre-workout snack.

INGREDIENTS FOR 1-2 SERVINGS

- ½ cup of plain yogurt
- ½ cup of plain water
- ½ cup of sliced mango
- 1 tbsp of sugar
- ¼ tsp of cardamom
- ¼ tsp cinnamon
- ¼ cup lime juice

METHOD

1. Pulse all the above ingredients in a blender until smooth (around 1 minute).

2. Pour into tall glasses or mason jars and serve chilled immediately.

NUTRITIONAL INFORMATION (Per Serving)

- Calories: 89.02 kcal
- Carbohydrate: 14.31 g
- Protein: 2.54 g
- Sodium: 30 mg
- Potassium: 185.67 mg
- Phosphorus: 67.88 mg
- Dietary Fiber: 0.77 g
- Fat: 2.05 g
- Sugar: 18 g

Breakfast Maple Sausage

COOKING TIME: 8 MINUTES

DESCRIPTION

If you are a meat lover, you will simply love this rich breakfast sausage recipe that is high in protein but low in phosphorus and potassium. You can also keep any leftovers of this for casseroles, omelets, and sandwiches.

INGREDIENTS FOR 12 SERVINGS

- 1 pound of pork, minced
- ½ pound lean turkey meat, ground
- ¼ tsp of nutmeg
- ½ tsp black pepper
- ¼ allspice
- 2 tbsp of maple syrup
- 1 tbsp of water

METHOD

1. Combine all the ingredients in a bowl.

2. Cover and place in the fridge for 3-4 hours.
3. Take the mixture and form it into small flat patties with your hand (around 10-12 patties).
4. Lightly grease a medium skillet with oil and shallow fry the patties over medium to high heat, until brown (around 4-5 minutes on each side).
5. Serve hot.

NUTRITIONAL INFORMATION (Per Serving)

- Calories: 53.85 kcal
- Carbohydrate: 2.42 g
- Protein: 8.5 g
- Sodium: 30.96 mg
- Potassium: 84.68 mg
- Phosphorus: 83.49 mg
- Dietary Fiber: 0.03 g
- Fat: 0.9 g
- Sugar: 2 g

Summer Veggie Omelette

COOKING TIME: 5 MINUTES

DESCRIPTION

This blend of summer veggies like zucchini, corn, and fresh onions helps you to realize how rich and nutrient-dense can omelette be. It's so filling that you won't need anything else other than a smoothie or tea for breakfast.

INGREDIENTS FOR 1-2 SERVINGS

- 4 large egg whites
- ¼ cup of sweet corn, frozen
- ⅓ cup of zucchini, grated
- 2 green onions, sliced
- 1 tbsp of cream cheese
- Kosher pepper

METHOD

1. Grease a medium pan with some cooking spray and add the onions, corn, and grated zucchini.

2. Saute for a couple of minutes until softened.
3. Beat the eggs together with the water, cream cheese, and pepper in a bowl.
4. Add the eggs into the veggie mixture in the pan, and let cook while moving the edges from inside to outside with a spatula, to allow raw egg to cook through the edges.
5. Flip the omelet with the help of a dish (placed over the pan and flipped upside down and then back to the pan).
6. Let sit for another 1-2 minutes.
7. Fold in half and serve.

NUTRITIONAL INFORMATION (Per Serving)

- Calories: 90 kcal
- Carbohydrate: 15.97 g
- Protein: 8.07 g
- Sodium: 227 mg
- Potassium: 244..24 mg
- Phosphorus: 45.32 mg

- Dietary Fiber: 0.88 g
- Fat: 2.44 g
- Sugar: 16.4 g

Raspberry Overnight Porridge

COOKING TIME: OVERNIGHT

DESCRIPTION

Many people dislike the texture of warm porridge alone but there is a delicious version of the good old porridge. In this recipe, the oats are soaked in almond milk overnight so they get soft and ready to enjoy the next morning.

INGREDIENTS FOR 1 SERVING

- ⅓ cup of rolled oats
- ½ cup almond milk
- 1 tbsp of honey
- 5-6 raspberries, fresh or canned and unsweetened

METHOD

1. Combine the oats, almond milk, and honey in a mason jar and place into the fridge overnight.
2. Serve the next morning with the raspberries on top.

NUTRITIONAL INFORMATION (Per Serving)

- Calories: 143.6 kcal
- Carbohydrate: 34.62 g
- Protein: 3.44 g
- Sodium: 77.88 mg
- Potassium: 153.25 mg
- Phosphorus: 99.3 mg
- Dietary Fiber: 7.56 g
- Fat: 3.91 g
- Sugar: 29.6 g

Lunch

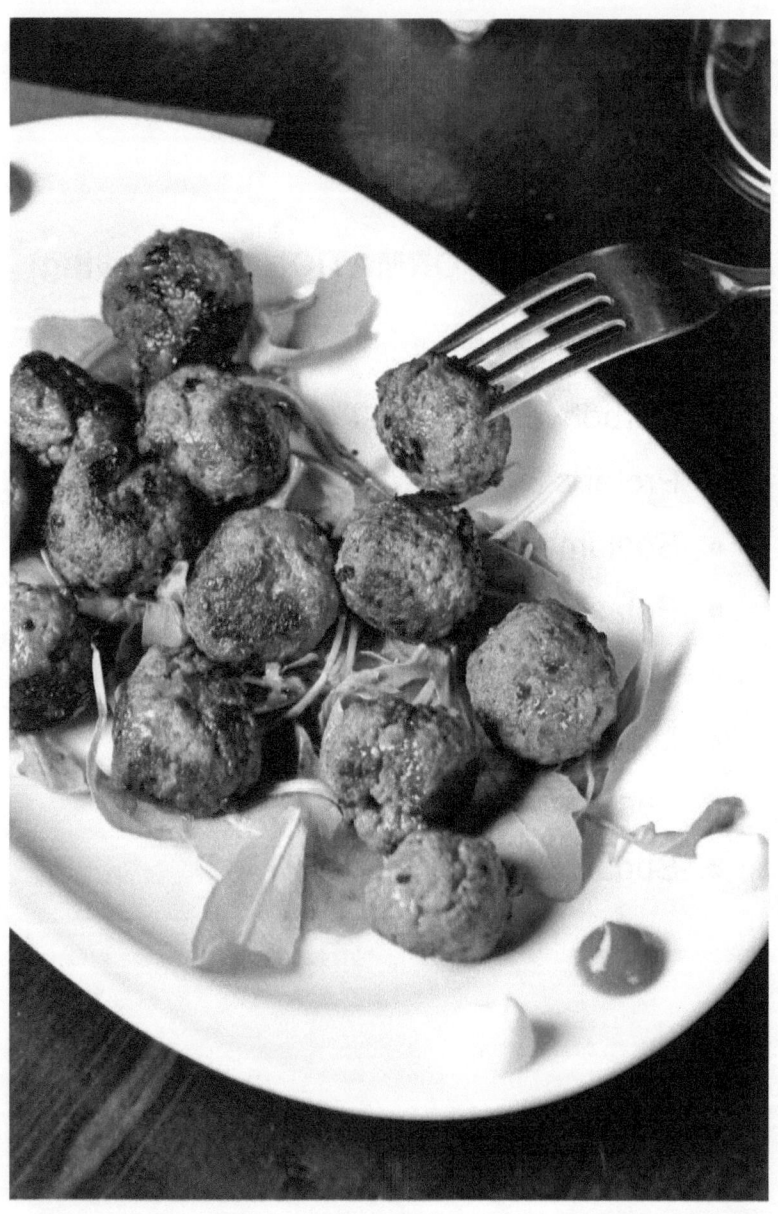

Light Beef Enchiladas

COOKING TIME: 15 MINUTES

DESCRIPTION

Enchiladas are a classic Mexican favorite for many; however, they can be hidden calorie and fat bombs. This recipe is much leaner yet equally delicious and, it has moderate to low amounts of potassium.

INGREDIENTS FOR 6 SERVING (12 enchiladas).

- 1 pound (around 650 grams) ground lean beef
- ½ cup shallots, chopped
- 1 clove of garlic
- 1 tsp of ground cumin
- ½ tsp cayenne pepper
- 1 can or small (200-gram jar) of enchilada sauce
- 12 corn tortillas
- A bit of low extra cheese on top (optional)

- Kosher pepper

METHOD

1. In a medium frying pan with 1 tsp of oil, brown the ground beef and the shallots (around 5-6 minutes).
2. Add the garlic and spices and toss to mix well. Cook until the meat will become brown and shallots will be soft and transparent. Add half of the enchilada sauce toss and cook for another 5 minutes.
3. Lightly toast the corn tortillas for 30-40 seconds on the toaster.
4. Distribute in each the remaining enchilada sauce and the ground beef mixture. Wrap and roll from one side to another to make enchiladas.
5. Sprinkle optionally a bit of grated cheddar cheese on top and place in the microwave for 1-2 minutes to melt the cheese and serve.

NUTRITIONAL INFORMATION (Per Serving)

- Calories: 286.70 kcal
- Carbohydrate: 30.75 g
- Protein: 26.3 g
- Sodium: 201.91 mg
- Potassium: 224.35 mg
- Phosphorus: 146.39 mg
- Dietary Fiber: 3.8 g
- Fat: 9 g
- Sugar: 3.5 g

Creamy Chicken with Cider

COOKING TIME: 25 MINUTES

DESCRIPTION

An easy 4-ingredient recipe that is full of flavor and is ready in under 30 minutes. Great as a family lunch on weekends or even as a hearty guest dish. It has a light gravy sauce for that extra dose of flavor.

INGREDIENTS FOR 8 SERVINGS

- 4 bone-in chicken breasts
- 2 tbsp of lightly salted butter
- ¾ cup apple cider vinegar
- ⅔ cup of rich unsweetened coconut milk or cream
- Kosher pepper

METHOD

1. Melt the butter in a skillet over medium heat.

2. Season the chicken with pepper and add to the skillet. Cook over low heat for approx. 20 minutes.
3. Remove the chicken from the heat and set it aside in a dish.
4. In the same skillet, add the cider and bring to a boil until most of it has evaporated.
5. Add the coconut cream and let cook for 1 minute until slightly thickened.
6. Pour the cider cream over the cooked chicken and serve.

NUTRITIONAL INFORMATION (Per Serving)

- Calories: 86.76 kcal
- Carbohydrate: 1.88 g
- Protein: 1.5 g
- Sodium: 93.52 mg
- Potassium: 74.65 mg
- Phosphorus: 36.54 mg
- Dietary Fiber: 0.1 g
- Fat: 8.21 g

- Sugar: 1.03 g

Easy and Fast Mac-n-Cheese

COOKING TIME: 8-10 MINUTES

DESCRIPTION

Mac-n-cheese is favorite soul food for kids and adults alike. It's not what we call "healthy" as it is loaded with a high amount of carbs but when on a renal diet, this is fine as it is very low in potassium and phosphorus.

INGREDIENTS FOR 4 SERVINGS

- 1 cup of dry elbow macaroni pasta
- ½ cup of mild cheddar cheese
- 3 cups of water
- 1 tsp of unsalted butter
- ½ tsp of dry mustard powder
- ½ tsp of paprika

METHOD

1. Boil the elbow macaroni in boiling water for 7-8 minutes (or until soft).
2. Drain all the water out and transfer it to the bowl.
3. Add the butter cheese, mustard, and paprika while the pasta is still hot, toss and serve.

NUTRITIONAL INFORMATION (Per Serving)

- Calories: 231.68 kcal
- Carbohydrate: 32.65 g
- Protein: 9.74 g
- Sodium: 107.25 mg
- Potassium: 29.52 mg
- Phosphorus: 159.93 mg
- Dietary Fiber: 0.12 g
- Fat: 7.2 g
- Sugar: 0.8 g

Italian Meatballs

COOKING TIME: 18 MINUTES

DESCRIPTION

Italian meatballs are renowned for their mild aromatic flavor and solid texture that blends ideally with a light tomato sauce. If you wish to try a low sodium alternative to this classic Italian dish, try this recipe.

INGREDIENTS FOR 12 SERVINGS

- 1.5 pounds of ground beef chuck,
- 2 eggs, beaten
- ½ cup of red onion, chopped
- ½ cup of rolled oat flakes
- ½ tsp of garlic salt
- 1 tsp of dried oregano
- 3 tbsp of parmesan cheese
- 1 tbsp of tomato paste
- ½ tsp of black pepper

METHOD

1. Preheat your oven at 375 F/190C.

2. Mix all the ingredients in a large bowl.
3. Shape into small balls (around 1 inch) and place on a Pyrex or baking sheet.
4. Bake for 15-17 minutes (or until they are fully cooked and slightly brown on the outside).
5. Remove from the oven and serve with a light tomato sauce or hot sauce and rice.

NUTRITIONAL INFORMATION (Per Serving)

- Calories: 133.12 kcal
- Carbohydrate: 5.8 g
- Protein: 14.4 g
- Sodium: 62.76 mg
- Potassium: 252.67 mg
- Phosphorus: 166.65 mg
- Dietary Fiber: 0.89 g
- Fat: 5.3 g
- Sugar: 0.53 g

Exotic Palabok

COOKING TIME: 12-15 MINUTES

DESCRIPTION

A delicious recipe from the Philippines that combines the flavors of rice noodles and shrimp.

INGREDIENTS FOR 6 SERVINGS

- 12 oz. rice noodles.
- 1 ½ cups of medium shrimp, peeled and deveined
- ⅔ cup white onion, chopped
- 1 spring onion, sliced
- 3 tbsp of canola oil
- 1 pound, lean ground turkey
- 2 cups firm tofu, chopped
- 2 packs of shrimp or ordinary gravy mix
- 5 hard-boiled eggs
- 1 lemon
- ½ cup of pork rinds (optional)

METHOD

1. Boil rice noodles until nice and soft. Keep aside.
2. Boil the peeled shrimp for 2-3 minutes in a pot with plain water.
3. In a wok or shallow pan, saute the garlic and onion with the oil. Add the ground turkey, tofu, and shrimps.
4. Dissolve the gravy mix in water or as per package instructions.
5. Combine the rice noodles, tofu, onions, and the gravy mix with ½ cup of pork rind (optional).
6. Slice the egg and lemons.
7. Serve with egg and lemons on top.

NUTRITIONAL INFORMATION (Per Serving)

- Calories: 305 kcal
- Carbohydrate: 39.14 g
- Protein: 17.6 g
- Sodium: 536 mg
- Potassium: 243.52 mg
- Phosphorus: 180.41 mg

- Dietary Fiber: 0.9 g
- Fat: 9 g
- Sugar: 0.24 g

Vegetarian Gobi Curry

COOKING TIME: 15 MINUTES

DESCRIPTION

An ethnic Indian recipe that comes from the Gobi desert area with a creamy and spicy flavor and texture that is a comfort for everyone. Vegetarians will love this recipe, as it's quite delicious and filling.

INGREDIENTS FOR 2 SERVINGS

- 2 cups of cauliflower florets
- 2 tbsp of unsalted butter
- 1 medium dry white onion, thinly chopped
- ½ cup of green peas(frozen if wish)
- 1 tsp of fresh ginger, chopped
- 1/2 tsp of turmeric
- 1 tsp of garam masala
- ¼ tsp cayenne pepper
- 1 tbsp of water

METHOD

1. Heat a skillet over medium heat with the butter and saute the onions until caramelized (golden brown).
2. Add the spices e.g. ginger, garam masala turmeric, and cayenne.
3. Add the cauliflower and the (frozen) peas and stir.
4. Add the water and cover with a lid. Reduce the heat to a low temperature and let cook covered for 10 minutes.
5. Serve with white rice.

NUTRITIONAL INFORMATION (Per Serving)

- Calories: 91.04 kcal
- Carbohydrate: 7.3 g
- Protein: 2.19 g
- Sodium: 39.38 mg
- Potassium: 209.58 mg
- Phosphorus: 42 mg
- Dietary Fiber: 3 g
- Fat: 6.4 g
- Sugar: 6 g

Marinated Shrimp and Pasta

COOKING TIME: 10 MINUTES

DESCRIPTION

A hearty recipe that combines shrimps, pasta, and various veggies for a burst of colors and flavors. A great pasta salad dish for lunch and guest food.

INGREDIENTS FOR 10 SERVINGS

- 12 oz. of three-colored penne pasta
- ½ pound of cooked shrimp
- ½ red bell pepper, diced
- ½ cup of red onion, chopped
- 3 stalks of celery
- 12 baby carrots, cut into thick slices
- 1 cup of cauliflower, cut into small round pieces
- ¼ cup of honey
- ¼ cup balsamic vinegar

- ½ tsp of black pepper
- ½ tsp garlic powder
- 1 tbsp of French mustard
- ¾ cup of olive oil

METHOD

1. Cook pasta for around 10 minutes (or according to packaged instructions).
2. While pasta is boiling, cut all your veggies and place into a large mixing bowl. Add the cooked shrimp.
3. In a mixing bowl, add the honey, vinegar, black pepper, garlic powder, and mustard.
4. While you whisk, slowly incorporate the oil and stir well.
5. Add in the drained pasta with the veggies and shrimp and gently combine everything.
6. Pour the liquid marinade over the pasta and veggies and toss to coat everything evenly.

7. Refrigerate for 3-5 hours before serving.
8. Serve chilled.

NUTRITIONAL INFORMATION (Per Serving)

- Calories: 256 kcal
- Carbohydrate: 41 g
- Protein: 6.55 g
- Sodium: 242.04 mg
- Potassium: 131.88 mg
- Phosphorus: 86.03 mg
- Dietary Fiber: 2.28 g
- Fat: 16.88 g
- Sugar: 12.6 g

Steak and Onion Sandwich

COOKING TIME: 8 MINUTES

DESCRIPTION

A rich steak sandwich that is very filling when you have to eat something good but don't have much time. Make this ahead for the next working day lunch or enjoy it fresh with the rest of your family.

INGREDIENTS FOR 4 SERVINGS

- 4 flank steaks (around 4 oz. each)
- 1 medium red onion, sliced
- 1 tbsp of lemon juice
- 1 tbsp of Italian seasoning
- 1 tsp of black pepper
- 1 tbsp of vegetable oil
- 4 sandwich/burger buns

METHOD

1. Wrap the steak with lemon juice, Italian seasoning, and pepper to taste. Cut into 4 pieces
2. Heat the vegetable oil in a medium skillet over medium heat.
3. Cook steaks for around 3 minutes on each side until you get a medium to well-done result. Take off and transfer onto a dish with absorbing paper.
4. In the same skillet, saute the onions until tender and transparent (around 3 minutes).
5. Cut the sandwich bun into half and place 1 piece of steak in each topped with the onions.
6. Serve or wrap with paper or foil and keep in the fridge for the next day.

NUTRITIONAL INFORMATION (Per Serving)

- Calories: 315.26 kcal
- Carbohydrate: 8.47 g
- Protein: 38.33 g

- Sodium: 266.24 mg
- Potassium: 238.2 mg
- Phosphorus: 364.25 mg
- Dietary Fiber: 0.76 g
- Fat: 13.22 g
- Sugar: 4.3 g

Zesty Crab Cakes

COOKING TIME: 6 MINUTES

DESCRIPTION

Crab cakes are a favorite dish in American seafood restaurants and are loved by kids and adults alike. If you like crab cakes, try this tasty recipe guilty-free as it is quite low on phosphorus and potassium.

INGREDIENTS FOR 6 SERVINGS

- 9 oz. (250 grams) of crab meat
- ⅓ cup green or red bell pepper, thinly chopped
- ⅓ cup low salt crackers, crushed
- ¼ cup low-fat mayonnaise
- 1 tbsp of dry mustard
- ½ tsp of pepper
- 2 tbsp of lemon juice
- ½ tsp of lemon zest
- 1 tsp of garlic powder
- 2 tbsp of vegetable oil

METHOD

1. Mix all the ingredients except for the oil until uniform. Divide into 6 flat patties (around 5 inches in diameter).
2. Heat the vegetable oil in the skillet and shallow fry the patties for 2-3 minutes on each side (or until golden brown).
3. Serve warm on a dish with absorbing paper.

NUTRITIONAL INFORMATION (Per Serving)

- Calories: 144.42 kcal
- Carbohydrate: 5.12 g
- Protein: 8.47 g
- Sodium: 212.31 mg
- Potassium: 195 mg
- Phosphorus: 127.42 mg
- Dietary Fiber: 1.02 g
- Fat: 9.2 g
- Sugar: 1.46 g

Stuffed Green Peppers

COOKING TIME: 36 MINUTES

DESCRIPTION

Green peppers are very delicious stuffed with rice and ground meat. This recipe calls for ground chicken or turkey and rice for a delicious yet light combo that is low in fat, potassium, and phosphorus.

INGREDIENTS FOR 6 SERVINGS

- 6 small to medium green peppers, seeds, and tops removed
- ½ pound of lean turkey or sausage meat
- ¼ cup red onions, chopped
- ¼ cup celery stalks, chopped
- 1 ½ cup of cooked white rice
- 2 tbsp of lemon juice
- 2 tbsp of Italian seasoning
- ½ tsp of black pepper
- ½ tsp of sugar
- 2 tbsp of vegetable oil

METHOD

1. Preheat the oven at 325F /180C.
2. Heat the vegetable oil in the pan.
3. Add in the pan the ground chicken, celery, onions, and cook until meat is become lightly brown (around 6-7 minutes).
4. Add all the remaining ingredients except peppers to the pan. Stir everything together and take off the heat.
5. Transfer and divide the mixture into the open green peppers. Place in a baking dish, cover, and bake for 30 minutes.
6. Serve hot.

NUTRITIONAL INFORMATION (Per Serving)

- Calories: 137.8 kcal
- Carbohydrate: 18.5 g
- Protein: 5.2 g
- Sodium: 182.65 mg
- Potassium: 251.36 mg
- Phosphorus: 64.97 mg

- Dietary Fiber: 3.5 g
- Fat: 5.2 g
- Sugar: 3.6 g

Dinner

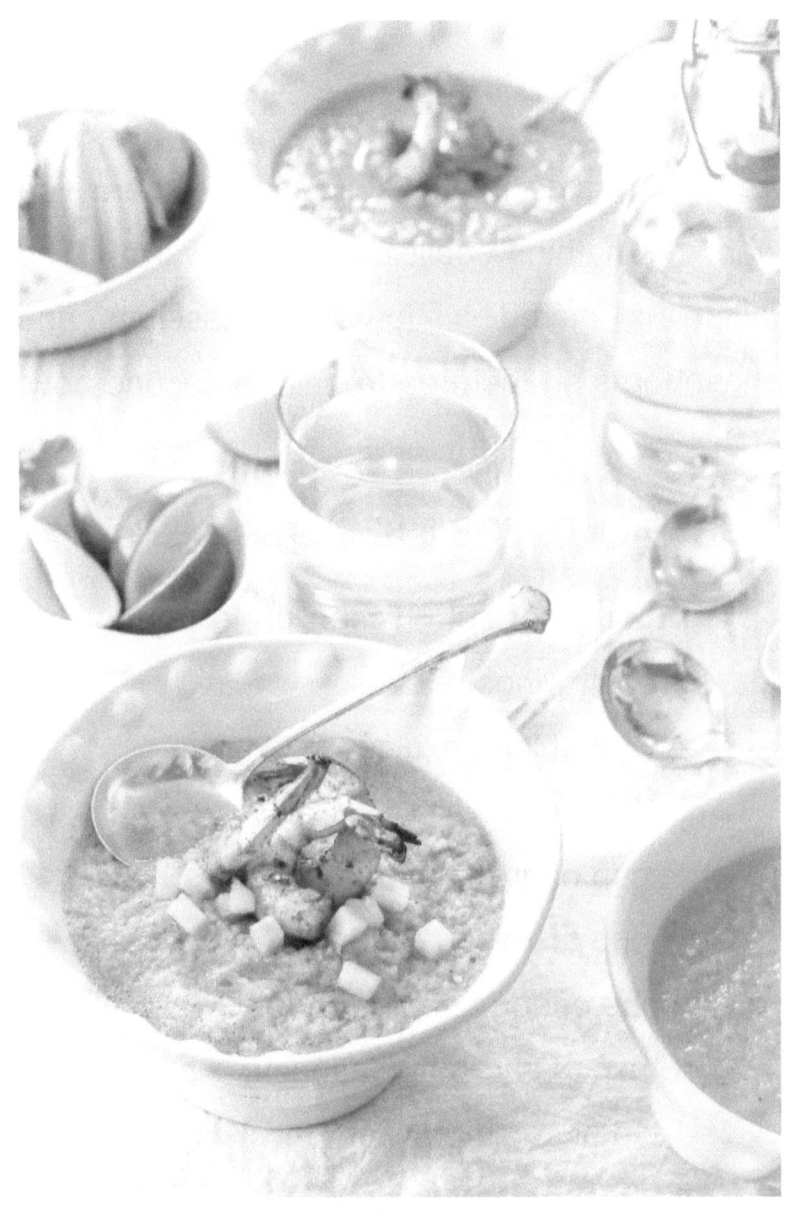

Chicken and Noodle Soup

COOKING TIME: 45 MINUTES

DESCRIPTION

A hearty recipe for the cold nights where you want something delicious and warm. The recipe is incredibly low in potassium and phosphorus so feel free to have a second bowl of this.

INGREDIENTS FOR 8 SERVINGS

- 1 pound of cut chicken parts e.g. thighs, breast, wings, etc.
- ¼ cup of lemon juice
- 3 ½ cups of water
- ½ cup of green pepper, diced
- ½ cup of celery, sliced
- 1 cup of egg noodles
- 1 tbsp of chicken seasoning
- 1 tsp of garlic powder
- 1 tsp of onion powder
- 1 tsp of red cayenne pepper

- 1 tsp of sugar
- 2 tbsp of vegetable oil

METHOD

1. Rub the chicken pieces with the lemon juice.
2. Combine chicken, water, chicken seasoning, and the rest of the spices with the sugar.
3. Bring to a boil and let cook for 30 minutes or until chicken is fully cooked and tender.
4. Add the pepper and noodles and cook for an extra 15 minutes.
5. Serve hot.

NUTRITIONAL INFORMATION (Per Serving)

- Calories: 66.45 kcal
- Carbohydrate: 6.92 g
- Protein: 1.29 g
- Sodium: 6.97 mg
- Potassium: 52.08 mg

- Phosphorus: 26.26 mg
- Dietary Fiber: 0.68 g
- Fat: 3.99 g
- Sugar: 0.5 g

Barbeque Turkey Cups

COOKING TIME: 12 MINUTES

DESCRIPTION

Try this delicious recipe of cups filled with turkey and barbeque sauce that is also very easy to make.

INGREDIENTS FOR 10 SERVINGS

- A 10 oz. package of frozen low-fat biscuits
- ¾ pounds of lean ground turkey breast
- ½ cup of mildly hot and spicy barbeque sauce
- 2 tsp of onion flakes
- ½ tsp of garlic powder
- 1 tbsp of vegetable oil

METHOD

1. Heat the oil in the skillet and add the ground turkey with the garlic powder, and cook until brown.

2. Add the onion flakes and the barbeque sauce and stir well.
3. Flatten each biscuit with a spatula and press into a muffin tin.
4. Distribute the barbeque/turkey mixture with a spoon to stuff each muffin.
5. Bake at 400 F/190 C in the oven for 10-12 minutes.

NUTRITIONAL INFORMATION (Per Serving)

- Calories: 178.15 kcal
- Carbohydrate: 16.92 g
- Protein: 11.28 g
- Sodium: 1660.32 mg
- Potassium: 178.3 mg
- Phosphorus: 203.57 mg
- Dietary Fiber: 0.71 g
- Fat: 7.15 g
- Sugar: 2.4 g

Low Sodium Green Bean Casserole

COOKING TIME: 30 MINUTES

DESCRIPTION

A holiday favorite dish made lighter with less sodium and fat yet still delicious and hearty with a bit of a slight crunch. You may cook this for dinner and then keep any leftovers for the next day.

INGREDIENTS FOR 8-10 SERVINGS

- 24 oz. of frozen green beans, thawed and cooked
- 1 red onion, chopped
- 2 garlic cloves, minced
- 1 cup of panko breadcrumbs
- ½ pound of fresh mushrooms, thinly sliced

- 3 cups of simple white/béchamel sauce (cooked with 4 tbsp of butter, 4 tbsp of flour and 4 cups of milk).

METHOD

1. Preheat your oven at 350F/180.
2. Melt in a skillet the butter and mix with breadcrumbs. Keep aside.
3. Saute the garlic and the onions in the remaining amount of butter until transparent and softened.
4. Add the sliced mushrooms and cook until soft (around 8 minutes).
5. In a lightly greased baking dish combine the green beans with the mushrooms and the cooked white sauce and stir well.
6. Top with the breadcrumbs and bake for 20-25 minutes or until golden brown on top.

NUTRITIONAL INFORMATION (Per Serving)

- Calories: 161.74 kcal

- Carbohydrate: 21.3 g
- Protein: 6.22 g
- Sodium: 322.53 mg
- Potassium: 233.37 mg
- Phosphorus: 140.3 mg
- Dietary Fiber: 5.53 g
- Fat: 6.94 g
- Sugar: 9.9 g

Marinated Mushrooms in the Broiler

COOKING TIME: 15 MINUTES

DESCRIPTION

Portobello mushrooms have a rich flavor and texture that almost resembles meat-especially if you cook them on the grill. You may try this broiler version that will be delicious.

INGREDIENTS FOR 5-6 SERVINGS

- 3 large Portobello mushrooms
- 1/3 cup of shallots, finely chopped
- 3 tbsp of balsamic vinegar
- ⅓ of brown sugar
- 3 tbsp of sesame oil
- 2 tbsp of low sodium soy sauce

METHOD

1. Wash the mushrooms, rinse and set aside.

2. Combine all the rest ingredients in a bowl to make a marinade. Add the mushrooms and let marinate in the fridge for at least 3 hours or overnight.
3. Place the mushrooms on a baking dish and cook in the broiler for 12-15 minutes.
4. Let the mushrooms rest for two minutes before serving.

NUTRITIONAL INFORMATION (Per Serving)

- Calories: 106.27 kcal
- Carbohydrate: 6.82 g
- Protein: 2.03 g
- Sodium: 212.98 mg
- Potassium: 196.75 mg
- Phosphorus: 74.8 mg
- Dietary Fiber: 1.18 g
- Fat: 8.58 g
- Sugar: 10.16 g

Italian Style Lamb Patties

COOKING TIME: 10 MINUTES

DESCRIPTION

A nice aromatic patty dish inspired by the flavors and aromas of the Italian and Mediterranean cuisine; oregano, feta, and garlic blend nicely with the lamb without overpowering its original taste.

INGREDIENTS FOR 12 SERVINGS

- 1 lb of ground lean lamb
- ½ cup of feta cheese, crumbled
- 1 clove of garlic, minced
- ½ tsp of dried oregano
- ½ tsp of crushed black pepper
- ¼ cup of white onion, chopped
- ¼ cup of panko breadcrumbs

METHOD

1. Combine the lamb with all the ingredients in a large bowl.

2. Shape into 4 patties of equal size (around ½ inch thick).
3. Heat a grilling and non-stick pan over medium heat with cooking spray.
4. Add the lamb patties and let them cook on high heat for nearly 5 minutes on each side. Ensure that the patties are no pink in the center by cutting one in half.
5. Serve

NUTRITIONAL INFORMATION (Per Serving)

- Calories: 118.39 kcal
- Carbohydrate: 2.1 g
- Protein: 7.5 g
- Sodium: 88.4 mg
- Potassium: 9.93 mg
- Phosphorus: 21.82 mg
- Dietary Fiber: 0.8 g
- Fat: 9.2 g
- Sugar: 0.33 g

Chicken with Jalapeno

COOKING TIME: 35 MINUTES

DESCRIPTION

An easy chicken recipe spiced up with the flavors of jalapeno pepper, nutmeg, and black pepper. The added chicken stock makes this extra juicy and flavorsome.

INGREDIENTS FOR 8 SERVINGS

- 2 ½ pounds of chicken pieces, skin and fat removed
- 1 onion, cut into rings
- 1 ½ cups of chicken stock
- 1/2 tsp of ground nutmeg
- 2 tsp of jalapeno peppers, chopped and seeds removed
- 2 tbsp of vegetable oil

METHOD

1. Heat the oil in the skillet and add the chicken pieces. Cook until brown and set aside.
2. Add the onion rings to the skillet with the oil and add the chicken stock, stirring occasionally.
3. Place the chicken pieces back to the pan. Add the pepper and nutmeg.
4. Cover the pan and let cook on low heat for 25-30 minutes.
5. Add the jalapeno peppers and cook for another two minutes.
6. Serve.

NUTRITIONAL INFORMATION (Per Serving)

- Calories: 256.18 kcal
- Carbohydrate: 1.79 g
- Protein: 31.1 g
- Sodium: 176.5 mg
- Potassium: 169.74 mg
- Phosphorus: 309.55 mg
- Dietary Fiber: 0.9 g

- Fat: 13.15 g
- Sugar: 0.5 g

Easy Mexican Soup

COOKING TIME: 35 MINUTES

DESCRIPTION

If you love Mexican flavors but don't want to go for something solid to ease your hunger, you may try this soup with corn and black beans that are so easy to make.

INGREDIENTS FOR 5-6 SERVINGS

- 1/3 cup of black beans (low fat)
- 1 can of sweet corn
- 1 tbsp of tomato paste
- 1 can of chicken bouillon soup
- 4 cups of water
- 2 boneless chicken thighs, skin and fat removed, chopped

METHOD

1. Mix all the ingredients in a pot and let cook on low heat for 30-35 minutes.
2. Serve hot.

NUTRITIONAL INFORMATION (Per Serving)

- Calories: 221.5 kcal
- Carbohydrate: 11.9 g
- Protein: 15 g
- Sodium: 323.98 mg
- Potassium: 337.65 mg
- Phosphorus: 170.8 mg
- Dietary Fiber: 2.26 g
- Fat: 13 g
- Sugar: 0.56 g

Seafood Casserole

COOKING TIME: 25 MINUTES

DESCRIPTION

A delicious casserole recipe made with crabmeat, tuna, and shrimps blended nicely with veggies for that extra flavor and crunch. Very low in fat, sodium, and phosphorus.

INGREDIENTS FOR 6 SERVINGS

- 1 cup of crab meat, boiled
- 1 cup of medium to small shrimp, boiled
- 4 tbsp of green pepper, diced
- ½ cup of frozen green peas
- 2 tbsp of green onions, chopped
- 1 cup of celery, sliced
- ½ cup of low-fat mayonnaise
- 1 cup of regular breadcrumbs

METHOD

1. Preheat the oven at 375F/180C.

2. Mix all the ingredients except for breadcrumbs in a mixing bowl. Stir and press lightly with a fork to make everything even.
3. Transfer the mixture into a greased casserole dish.
4. Place the breadcrumbs on top.
5. Bake for 25-20 minutes.

NUTRITIONAL INFORMATION (Per Serving)

- Calories: 225.1 kcal
- Carbohydrate: 18.17 g
- Protein: 16.4 g
- Sodium: 609.55 mg
- Potassium: 213.49 mg
- Phosphorus: 211.39 mg
- Dietary Fiber: 2.6 g
- Fat: 9.4 g
- Sugar: 1.66 g

Beef and Veggie Soup

COOKING TIME: 50 MINUTES

DESCRIPTION

This soup recipe will remind you of the classic Sunday beef stew, as the ingredients are nearly the same but on a soup version. A lovely soup for the entire family.

INGREDIENTS FOR 8 SERVING

- 1 pound of beef pieces, for stew
- 2/3 cup of white onion, sliced
- ½ cup of frozen green peas
- ⅓ cup carrot, diced
- ½ of frozen corn kernels
- 3 ½ cups of water
- ½ tsp of dried basil
- ½ tsp of thyme
- 2 tbsp of olive oil

METHOD

1. Grease the bottom of a large pot with olive oil and place the onions with all the fresh veggies, and saute for 3-4 minutes.
2. Add the frozen veggies, the meat and let simmer on low heat for 45-50 minutes.
3. Serve hot.

NUTRITIONAL INFORMATION (Per Serving)

- Calories: 108.3 kcal
- Carbohydrate: 9.36 g
- Protein: 3.24 g
- Sodium: 233.57 mg
- Potassium: 167.97 mg
- Phosphorus: 43.42 mg
- Dietary Fiber: 1.4 g
- Fat: 6.7 g
- Sugar: 0.9 g

Pepper Linguini Pasta

COOKING TIME: 12 MINUTES

DESCRIPTION

A simple yet delicious recipe made with thin linguini pasta and roasted bell peppers for a bit of kick. The thyme and the butter add an extra dimension of flavor to this dish.

INGREDIENTS FOR 7-8 SERVINGS

- 1 pack (16 0.z) of uncooked linguine pasta.
- ¾ cup of lightly salted butter
- 2 tbsp of fresh thyme
- 5 roasted red bell peppers, roughly chopped
- 3 cloves of garlic, minced
- 2 tbsp of olive oil

METHOD

1. Fill half of a large pot with water and add the linguini pasta and olive oil. Allow

cooking for 8-10 minutes (until softened). Drain and keep aside.
2. Heat two tbsp of butter in a pan over medium heat. Add the minced garlic and cook until golden brown. Add the rest of the butter, thyme, and roasted bell peppers. Let cook until everything is heated evenly (around 2-3 minutes).
3. Serve the pepper sauce over the boiled pasta.

NUTRITIONAL INFORMATION (Per Serving)

- Calories: 407.75 kcal
- Carbohydrate: 50.11 g
- Protein: 8.78 g
- Sodium: 143.5 mg
- Potassium: 100.98 mg
- Phosphorus: 221.25 mg
- Dietary Fiber: 6.85 g
- Fat: 22.6 g
- Sugar: 1.3 g

Desserts

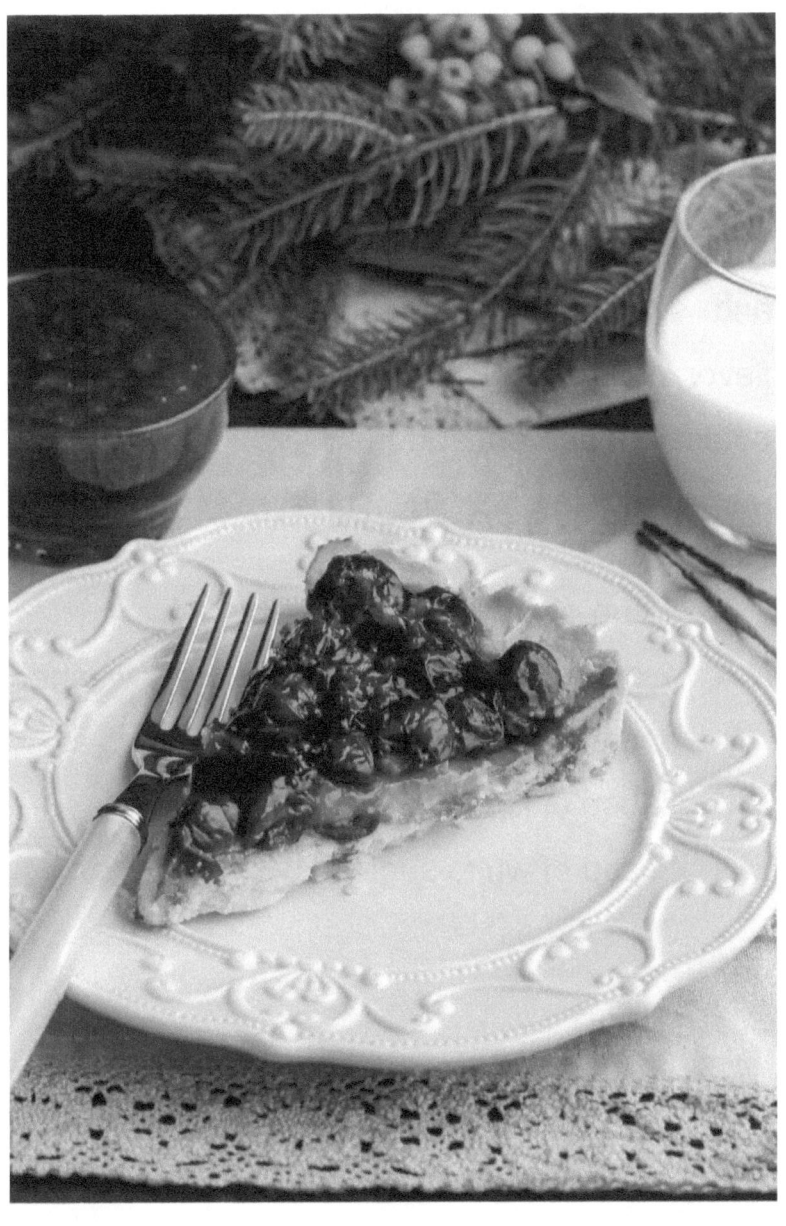

Dessert Cocktail

COOKING TIME: 1 MINUTE

DESCRIPTION

A rich dessert and non-alcoholic cocktail made of forest fruits like cranberries and strawberries and sweetened with sugar, despite its rich flavor; it has 100 calories and is very low in potassium and phosphorus.

INGREDIENTS FOR 4 SERVINGS

- 1 cup of cranberry juice
- 1 cup of fresh ripe strawberries, washed and hull removed
- 2 tbsp of lime juice
- ¼ cup of white sugar
- 8 ice cubes

METHOD

1. Combine all the ingredients in a blender until smooth and creamy.

2. Pour the liquid into chilled tall glasses and serve cold.

NUTRITIONAL INFORMATION (Per Serving)

- Calories: 92 kcal
- Carbohydrate: 23.5 g
- Protein: 0.5 g
- Sodium: 3.62 mg
- Potassium: 103.78 mg
- Phosphorus: 17.86 mg
- Dietary Fiber: 0.84 g
- Fat: 0.17 g
- Sugar: 23.7 g

Baked Egg Custard

COOKING TIME: 30 MINUTES

DESCRIPTION

A lovely and traditional egg custard recipe that you can enjoy on its own or as an extra in other dessert recipes. Very easy to make with just 5 ingredients.

INGREDIENTS FOR 4 SERVINGS

- 2 medium eggs, at room temperature
- ¼ cup of semi-skimmed milk
- 3 tbsp of white sugar
- ½ tsp of nutmeg
- 1 tsp of vanilla extract

METHOD

1. Preheat your oven at 375 F/180C
2. Mix all the ingredients in a mixing bowl and beat with a hand mixer for a few seconds until creamy and uniform.

3. Pour the mixture into lightly greased muffin tins.
4. Bake for 25-30 minutes or until the knife, you place inside, comes out clean.

NUTRITIONAL INFORMATION (Per Serving)

- Calories: 96.56 kcal
- Carbohydrate: 10.5 g
- Protein: 3.5 g
- Sodium: 37.75 mg
- Potassium: 58.19 mg
- Phosphorus: 58.76 mg
- Dietary Fiber: 0.06 g
- Fat: 2.91 g
- Sugar: 1.8 g

Gumdrop Cookies

COOKING TIME: 12 MINUTES

DESCRIPTION

A lively cookie recipe that is great for kids and will remind your childhood. If you have an upcoming kid's party, these cookies will be devoured in seconds.

INGREDIENTS FOR 25 SERVINGS

(50 cookies)

- ½ cup of spreadable unsalted butter
- 1 medium egg
- 1 cup of brown sugar
- 1 ⅔ cups of all-purpose flour, sifted
- ¼ cup of milk
- 1 tsp vanilla
- 1 tsp of baking powder
- 15 large gumdrops, chopped finely

METHOD

1. Preheat the oven at 400F/195C.

2. Combine the sugar, butter, and egg until creamy.
3. Add the milk and vanilla and stir well.
4. Combine the flour with the baking powder in a different bowl. Incorporate to the sugar, butter mixture, and stir.
5. Add the gumdrops and place the mixture in the fridge for half an hour.
6. Drop the dough with tablespoonful into a lightly greased baking or cookie sheet.
7. Bake for 10-12 minutes or until golden brown.

NUTRITIONAL INFORMATION (Per Serving)
- Calories: 102.17 kcal
- Carbohydrate: 16.5 g
- Protein: 0.86 g
- Sodium: 23.42 mg
- Potassium: 45 mg
- Phosphorus: 32.15 mg
- Dietary Fiber: 0.13 g
- Fat: 4 g

- Sugar: 2.24 g

Pound Cake with Pineapple

COOKING TIME: 50 MINUTES

DESCRIPTION

An old school cake recipe accentuated with the exotic flavors of pineapple for that sweet and slightly sour taste. Bake this and enjoy the same day or up to 5 days after baking.

INGREDIENTS FOR 24 SERVINGS

(1 cake/24 slice).

- 3 cups of all-purpose flour, sifted
- 3 cups of sugar
- 1 ½ cups of butter
- 6 whole eggs and 3 egg whites
- 1 tsp of vanilla extract
- 1 10.oz can of pineapple chunks, rinsed and crushed (keep the juice aside).

For the glaze

- 1 cup of sugar
- 1 stick of unsalted butter or margarine

- Reserved juice from the pineapple

METHOD

1. Preheat the oven at 350F/180C.
2. Beat the sugar and the butter with a hand mixer until creamy and smooth.
3. Slowly add the eggs (one or two every time) and stir well after pouring each egg.
4. Add the vanilla extract, follow up with the flour and stir well.
5. Add the drained and chopped pineapple.
6. Pour the mixture into a greased cake tin and bake for 45-50 minutes.
7. In a small saucepan, combine the sugar with the butter and pineapple juice. Stir every few seconds and bring to boil. Cook until you get creamy to a thick glaze consistency.
8. Pour the glaze over the cake while still hot.
9. Let cook for at least 10 seconds and serve.

NUTRITIONAL INFORMATION (Per Serving)

- Calories: 407.4 kcal
- Carbohydrate: 79 g
- Protein: 4.25 g
- Sodium: 118.97 mg
- Potassium: 180.32 mg
- Phosphorus: 66.37 mg
- Dietary Fiber: 2.25 g
- Fat: 16.48 g
- Sugar: 18.6 g

Apple Crunch Pie

COOKING TIME: 35 MINUTES

DESCRIPTION

A lovely twist to the classic apple pie recipe with an added crunch on top of the apples. Made just with 6 ingredients and under 40 minutes. Feel free to serve this with a scoop of vanilla ice cream.

INGREDIENTS FOR 8 SERVINGS

- 4 large tart apples, peeled, seeded, and sliced
- ½ cup of white all-purpose flour
- ⅓ cup margarine
- 1 cup of sugar
- ¾ cup of rolled oat flakes
- ½ tsp of ground nutmeg

METHOD

1. Preheat the oven to 375F/180C.

2. Place the apples over a lightly greased square pan (around 7 inches).
3. Mix the rest of the ingredients in a medium bowl and spread the batter over the apples.
4. Bake for 30-35 minutes or until the top crust has gotten golden brown.
5. Serve hot.

NUTRITIONAL INFORMATION (Per Serving)

- Calories: 261.9 kcal
- Carbohydrate: 47.2 g
- Protein: 1.5 g
- Sodium: 81 mg
- Potassium: 123.74 mg
- Phosphorus: 35.27 mg
- Dietary Fiber: 2.81 g
- Fat: 7.99 g
- Sugar: 18.65 g

Easy Chocolate Pie Shell

COOKING TIME: 30 MINUTES

DESCRIPTION

Do you wish to make an easy shell for your chocolate or custard pie from scratch? This recipe requires just 2 ingredients and it's so easy that even a kid can make it.

INGREDIENTS FOR 6 SERVINGS
(6 servings/one empty pie crust)

- 3 cups of cocoa rice Krispies, crushed
- ½ stick of unsalted butter, melted

METHOD

1. Place crushed cocoa Krispies in a bowl with the melted butter. Mix well with a spatula.
2. Spray an 8-9 inch pie pan with some low-calorie cooking spray
3. Press the mixture into the pan and even out with a spatula.

4. Let sit and chill for at least 30 minutes in the fridge prior to filling it with chocolate or vanilla pudding.

NUTRITIONAL INFORMATION (Per Serving)

- Calories: 113.1 kcal
- Carbohydrate: 11.6 g
- Protein: 0.88 g
- Sodium: 122.98 mg
- Potassium: 17.3 mg
- Phosphorus: 18.23 mg
- Dietary Fiber: 0.04 g
- Fat: 7.82 g
- Sugar: 8 g

Strawberry and Mint Sorbet

COOKING TIME: 1 MINUTE

DESCRIPTION

Sorbets are probably one of the tangiest and refreshing desserts as they are fruity while containing low amounts of fat. Make this and enjoy it alone or with other desserts.

INGREDIENTS FOR 3-4 SERVINGS

- ¼ cup of white sugar
- 1 cup of frozen or fresh, sliced strawberries
- 1 tbsp of lime juice
- ¼ cup of water
- 1 ¼ cup of crushed ice
- A few mint leaves

METHOD

1. Pulse and crush the ice in a heavy-duty blender.

2. Add the remaining ingredients and raise the speed to crush until no lumps of ice are left.
3. Optionally add a few mint leaves for garnishing.

NUTRITIONAL INFORMATION (Per Serving)

- Calories: 93.34 kcal
- Carbohydrate: 32 g
- Protein: 0.33 g
- Sodium: 2.12 mg
- Potassium: 113.02 mg
- Phosphorus: 10.24 mg
- Dietary Fiber: 1.56 g
- Fat: 0.067 g
- Sugar: 11.06 g

Easy Chocolate Fudge

COOKING TIME: 10 MINUTES

DESCRIPTION

An old school fudge recipe will be easy to cook with just five ingredients and ready in 20 minutes (including cooling time). Make this ahead and keep for up two weeks at room temperature.

INGREDIENTS FOR 12 SERVINGS

- ⅔ cup of half and half cream
- 1 cup of white granulated sugar
- 1 cups of semi-sweet chocolate chip cookies
- 1 cup of mini marshmallows
- 1 tsp of vanilla extract

METHOD

1. Grease with cooking spray a square pie pan (around 9 inches).

2. Mix the half-and-half cream with the sugar in a medium saucepan. Bring to a boil and adjust to medium heat.
3. Take off the heat and add the chocolate chips, the marshmallows, and the vanilla extract. Stir well with a spatula until everything will be melted.
4. Quickly transfer the mixture into the pie pan. Let cool for at least 10 minutes and cut into square pieces, around 3x2" each. This will make 18-20 pieces.

NUTRITIONAL INFORMATION (Per Serving)

- Calories: 52.4 kcal
- Carbohydrate: 17.58 g
- Protein: 3.18 g
- Sodium: 153.47 mg
- Potassium: 100.52 mg
- Phosphorus: 38.63 mg
- Dietary Fiber: 1.35 g
- Fat: 21.3 g
- Sugar: 32.83 g

High Protein Vanilla Cookies

COOKING TIME: 12 MINUTES

DESCRIPTION

A delicious recipe with vanilla aromas amplified with extra whey protein powder and oatmeal for a bit of extra fiber. Enjoy and keep up to two weeks at room temperature.

INGREDIENTS FOR 12 SERVINGS (24 cookies)

- ¾ cup of all-purpose flour
- ½ cup of oatmeal
- ½ cup of whey protein powder
- ¾ cups of brown sugar
- 1 egg
- 1 tsp of vanilla extract
- 1 tsp of baking soda
- 3 tbsp of margarine

METHOD

1. Preheat your oven at 325F/165C
2. Beat with the mixer the butter and the brown sugar.
3. Add the egg and the vanilla extract
4. Combine all the other ingredients until smooth (the mixture will be a tad drier than most cookie doughs).
5. Roll the batter with your hands into 1"balls.
6. Lightly grease a baking sheet and the cookie balls.
7. Bake for 10-12 minutes.

NUTRITIONAL INFORMATION (Per Serving)

- Calories: 292.95 kcal
- Carbohydrate: 29.1 g
- Protein: 35.1 g
- Sodium: 173.07 mg
- Potassium: 291.27 mg
- Phosphorus: 629.72 mg
- Dietary Fiber: 4.67 g
- Fat: 1.51 g

- Sugar: 21 g

Easy Pumpkin Pudding

COOKING TIME: 8-10 MINUTES

DESCRIPTION

If you love the festive flavors of pumpkin but don't want to get in the fuss of making a pumpkin pie, you can try this delicious and incredibly easy pumpkin pudding with just 5 ingredients.

INGREDIENTS FOR 4 SERVINGS

- 3 oz. instant vanilla pudding mix powder
- 1 cup almond milk
- ½ cup of pumpkin puree
- 1 tsp of pumpkin spice mix
- 1 scoop of vanilla flavored protein powder

METHOD

1. In a saucepan, mix the pudding mix and the almond milk.

2. Bring to a boil and reduce the heat as soon as the pudding has started to thicken.
3. Take off the heat and mix in the pumpkin puree, the pumpkin spice, and the protein powder. Stir well.
4. Transfer into a big glass bowl, let chill, and cover with plastic wrap. Refrigerate for at least 5 hours before serving.

NUTRITIONAL INFORMATION (Per Serving)

- Calories: 120.32 kcal
- Carbohydrate: 22.8 g
- Protein: 5.49 g
- Sodium: 370.66 mg
- Potassium: 84.44 mg
- Phosphorus: 164.57 mg
- Dietary Fiber: 0.9 g
- Fat: 0.84 g
- Sugar: 21.5 g

Conclusion

Renal diet may seem restricting for many, but in reality, there are plenty of low sodium, low phosphorus, and low potassium options to try out and we have proven it with this recipe book.

Keep in mind that we have included roughly the levels of all these minerals in every recipe separately and therefore, you will have to calculate the total amounts you consume each day with all your daily meals.

Generally, most experts suggest up to 2700 mg of potassium and phosphorus per day for patients at the first two stages of the renal disease while those at a more advanced stage should aim to consume up to 2000mg of these two minerals (each) per day to avoid dialysis. Since most of the recipes featured in this e-book contain up to 250 mg of potassium and phosphorus respectively, you can eat your breakfast, lunch, and dinner without worrying about crossing your daily limits.

Don't forget to do regular doctor check-ups to monitor your progress.

Please always consult with your family doctor or nutritionist before your diet plan formation.

Thanks for your attention!

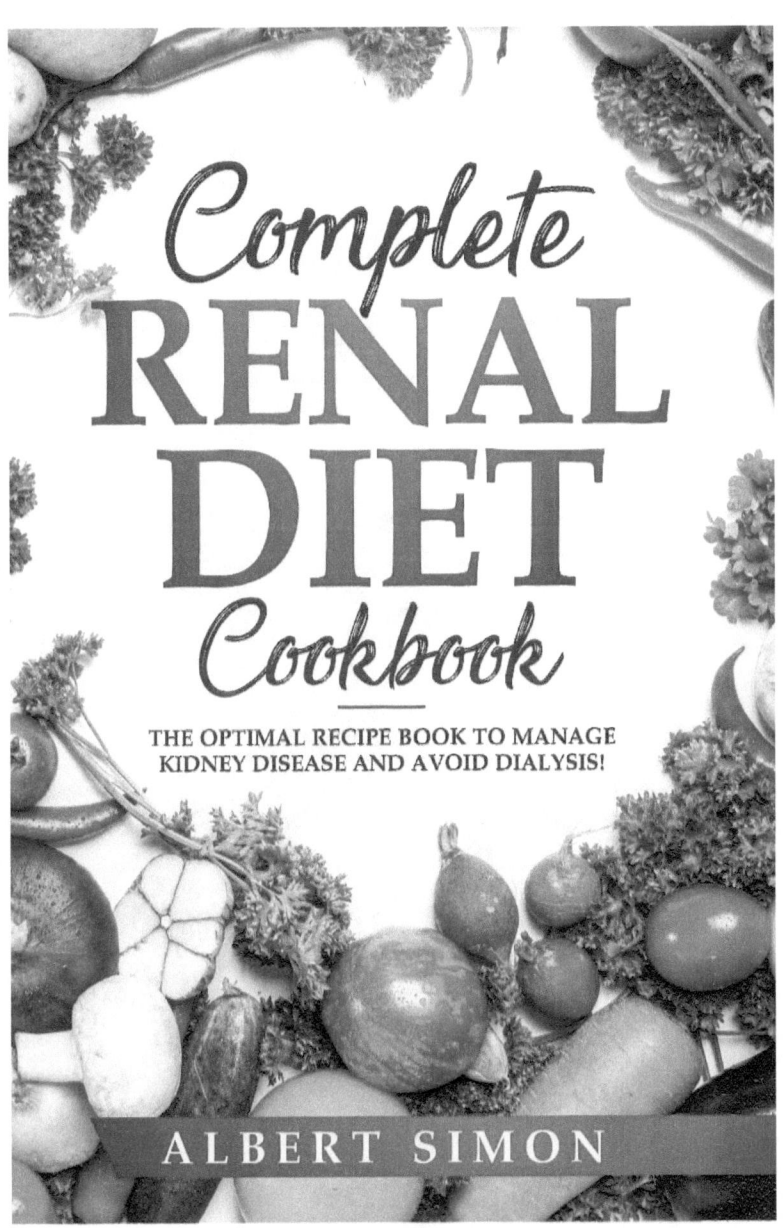

Complete Renal Diet Cookbook

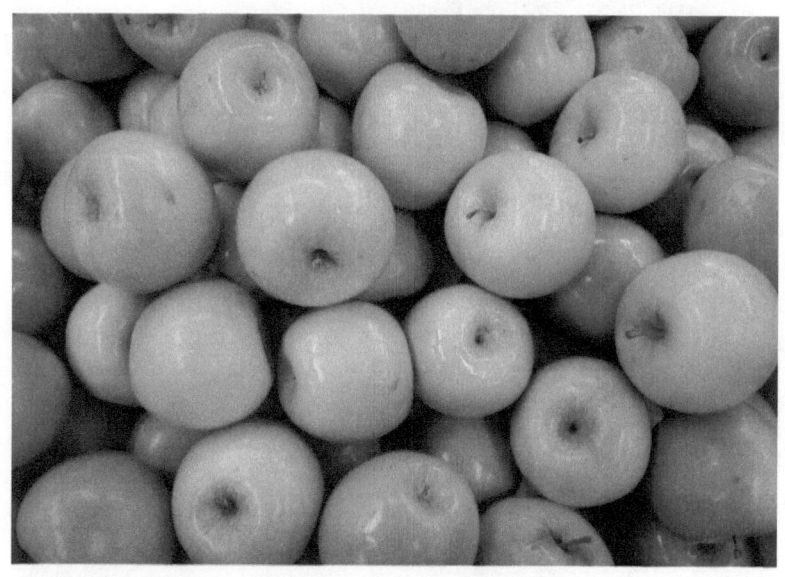

THE OPTIMAL RECIPE BOOK TO MANAGE KIDNEY DISEASE AND AVOID DIALYSIS!

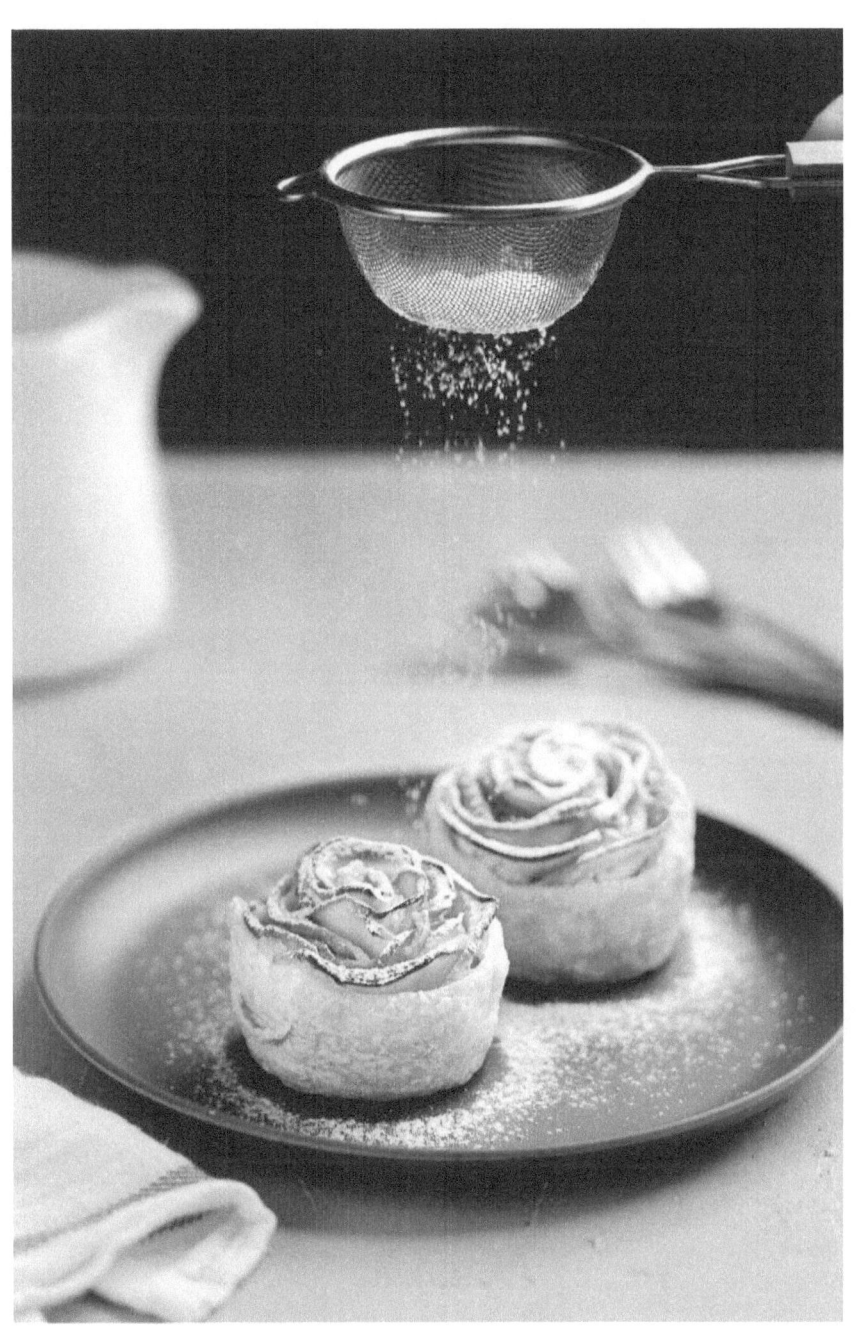

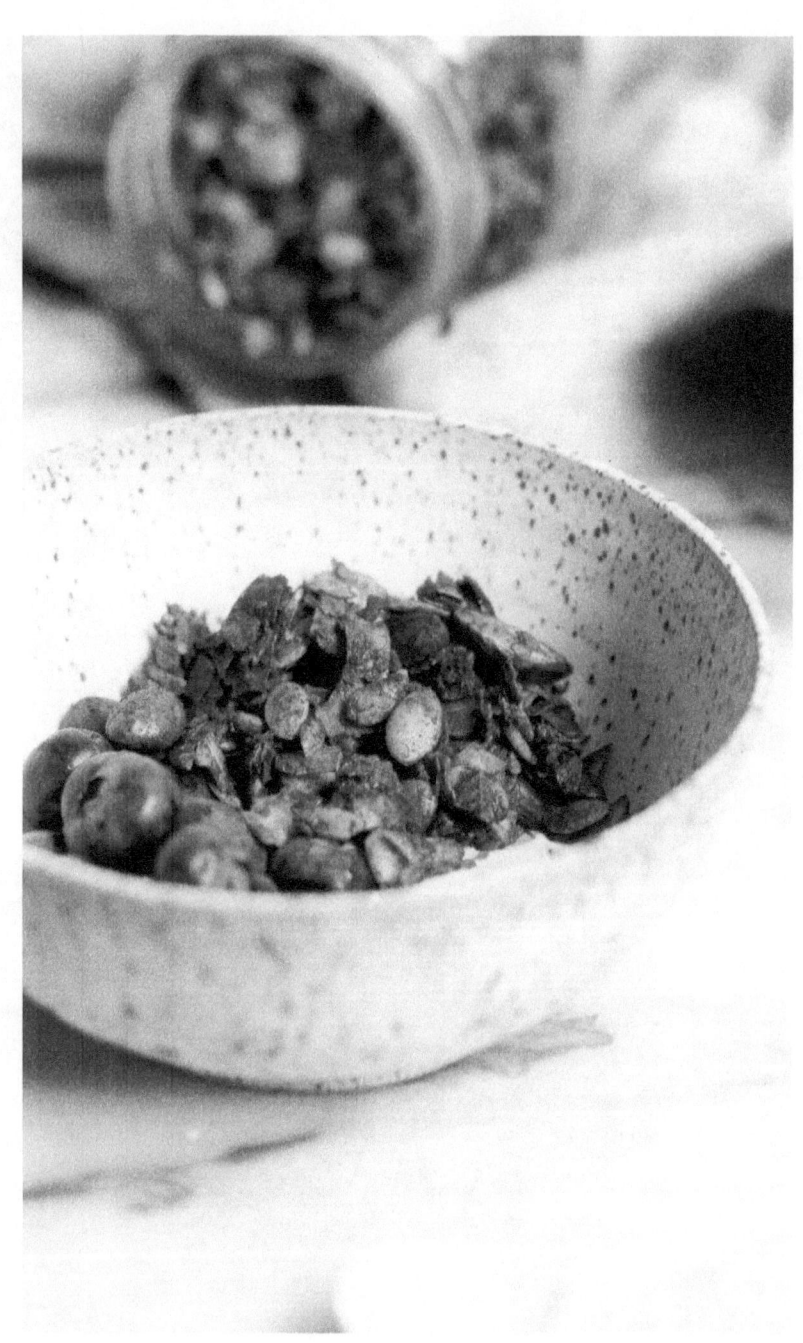

TABLE OF CONTENTS

Introduction 149
What is Kidney Disease? Main Causes 150
The History of Renal Diet 156
Why Do You Need Renal Diet? 157
The Explanation of Key Diet Words 159
What Food to Eat and What to Avoid? 165
List of Juices and Drinks in Renal Diet 171
Frequently Asked Questions 173
Recipes 177
   Breakfast 178
      Egg White and Pepper Omelette 179
      Blueberry Smoothie Bowl 181
      Turkey Breakfast Sausage 183
      Italian Apple Fritters 185
      Tofu and Mushroom Scramble 187
      Sunny Pineapple Breakfast Smoothie ... 189
      Puff Oven Pancakes 191
      Savory Muffins with Protein 194
      Tex-Mex Sausage 197
      European Pancakes 199
      Multigrain Warm Porridge 202

    Puffy French Toast 204
Lunch... 206
    Couscous with Veggies 207
    Mexican Steak Tacos 210
    Beer Pork Ribs 213
    Crispy Lemon Chicken 215
    Mexican Chorizo Sausage 218
    Eggplant Casserole 221
    Easy Cilantro Cod 224
    Light Greek Soutzoukakia 226
    Pizza with Chicken & Pesto 228
    Easy Egg Salad 231
    Shrimp Quesadilla 233
    Grilled Corn on the Cob 236
Dinner 238
    Creamy Crab Soup 239
    Broccoli Onion Latkes 242
    Glazed Carrots 245
    Slow Cooker Chicken 247
    Syrian Style Lamb Kafta 249
    Spicy Lime Shrimp 251
    Pasta Shells with Peas and Bacon 254

- Buffalo Chicken Wings 258
- Cauliflower and Apple Soup 261
- Mapo's Tofu and Pork 264
- Lemon Orzo Salad 267
- Sausage Stuffed Jalapenos 269
- Desserts 271
  - Raspberry Mousse 272
  - Honey Ginger Cookies 274
  - Honey Baked Pear 277
  - Watermelon Sorbet 279
  - Aunt Tula's Carrot Cake 281
- Conclusion 284

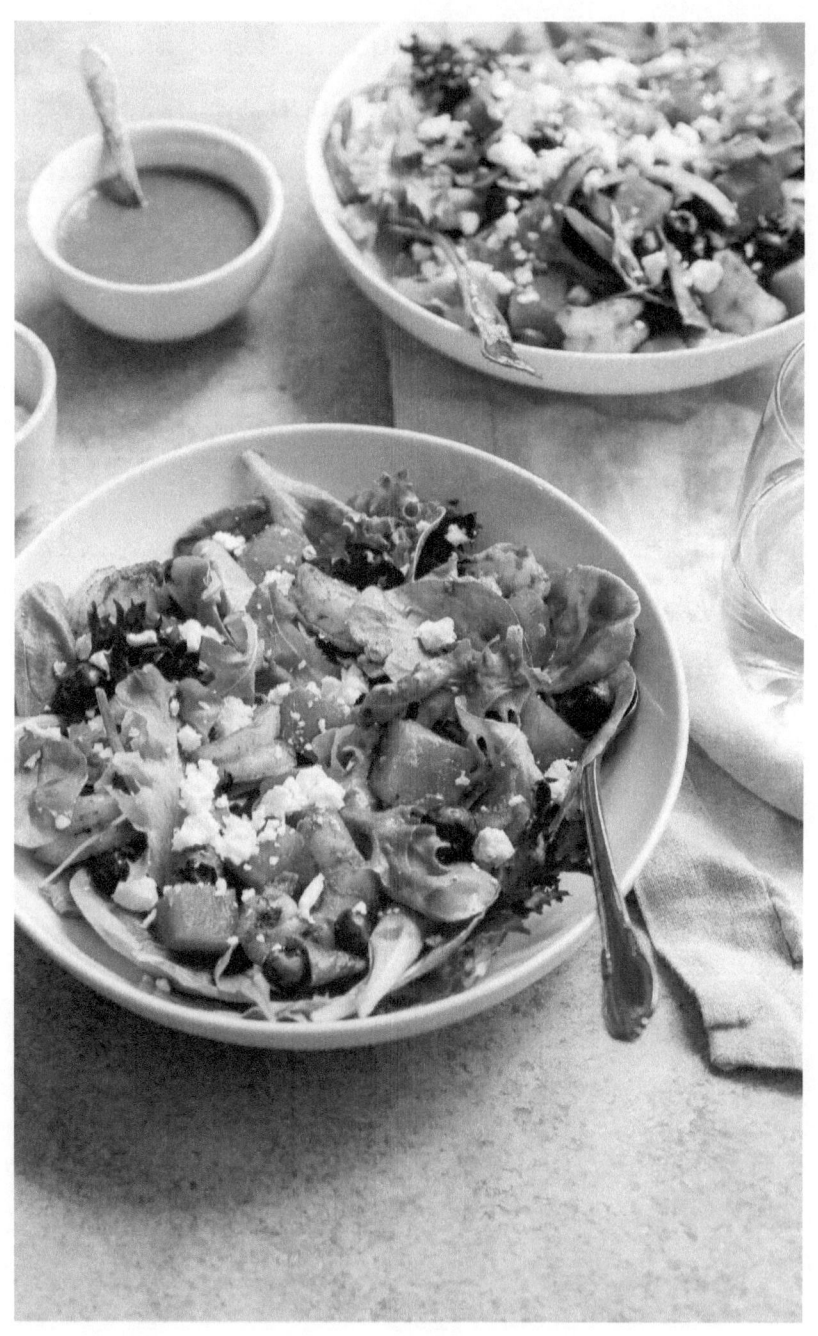

Introduction

Have you been diagnosed with renal disease? If yes, and your doctor has advised you some general diet guidelines on what to eat and what to avoid, maybe you still wondering about some details and recipes to try out while being on a renal diet.

Being in the first stages of renal damage you should follow a Renal diet correctly as it can slow down the progression of the disease and help you avoid dialysis.

In this book, we aim to tackle all your main concerns regarding renal diet and give you detailed recipes that follow all renal diet specifics, so keep on reading.

What is Kidney Disease? Main Causes

Kidney disease or in other words "renal disease" and "kidney damage" is a health condition where the kidneys are unable to function in a healthy and proper manner.

How kidneys work and what is their role in our systems?

Kidneys are vital organs located in our lower body backs (around the ribcage area) that are responsible for filtering out the toxins and junk out of our bloodstream through the urine. To preserve the balance in our systems, kidneys help regulate salts and minerals circulating in our bodies such as sodium, phosphorus, and potassium. Our kidneys also release hormonal compounds that help regulate blood pressure, build new red blood cells, and maintain the health of bones and connective tissue.

Kidney disease, in this case, is a chronic condition (CKD) where the kidneys fail gradually to do their normal job. Chronic kidney disease typically develops in 5 stages. Each stage is measured by a formula called Glomerular Filtration Rate (GFR) which is calculated by several variables like age, race, gender, and the amount of serum creatinine in the urine. The higher this protein is in the system, the more progressed the stage of renal disease will be. Here is a brief snapshot of each stage.

Stage 1: considered normal or high risk of developing CKD. The GFR falls > 90 ml/min.

Stage 2: considered as mild CKD. The GFR falls in the range of 60-89 ml/min.

Stage 3: Moderate CKD which ranges from 45-59 ml/min.

Stage 4: Severe Chronic Kidney disease. Rates fall between 15-29 ml/min.

Stage 5: Final/end-stage of the renal disease which calls for surgery or dialysis. Also known as End-Stage Renal Disease (ESRD). The GFR levels, in this case, fall below 15 mL/min.

Now, in regards to the actual causes or risk factors that may contribute to the formation of disease, studies have indicated the following conditions:

Diabetes. Diabetes is probably the No.1 cause of renal disease as the increased blood glucose in the bloodstream can actually ruin blood vessels inside the kidneys.

Heart disease. Heart disease has also been found to have a negative association with CKD. Those with chronic heart problems, in particular, have a higher probability of developing the renal disease as well.

Elevated blood pressure. Abnormally high blood pressure, similarly to diabetes can ruin the delicate blood vessels inside the kidneys and make them function poorly as a result.

Genetic History of Renal Disease. If any of your family members and especially parents and grandparents have already developed the disease, there is a higher risk you are going to develop it too. If any of your family members has kidney disease, it would be wise to get tested too and encourage other family members to do the same.

In addition to the above common causes, autoimmune disorders like Lupus and nephrotic syndrome can increase the risk of developing renal disease. Also, urinary problems and certain medications e.g. diuretics or antibiotics, as well as illegal drugs, can interfere with the normal function of the kidneys and cause damage. For this reason, it would be wise to consult your doctor and take drugs for other conditions e.g. diabetes that does not harm your kidneys as a side effect.

The problem with the disease is that it often comes with little or no symptoms at all, especially during the first stages. You may experience the following symptoms, but these could also be a sign of another condition:

- Less frequent urination
- A very little amount of urine
- Sudden and unexplained pauses in breath
- Nausea
- Chest or back pain
- Drowsiness and dizziness
- Fatigue/feeling tired more than before
- Confusion
- Loss of balance
- Swelling in the face, ankles, feet, and hands
- Poor appetite

In extreme cases and stages e.g. renal failure, seizures and coma may also occur. However, it would be best for you to avoid looking solely for these symptoms and get tested to find out whether you have a chronic disease or not.

The History of Renal Diet

A renal diet is a medical treatment measure that has been followed for over three decades to stop the progression of renal disease. The vast majority of doctors and hospitals advise their patients to follow a renal diet program for this purpose.

Along with certain prescribed medications and lifestyle changes, renal disease has been proven to be a valuable weapon against the need for hemodialysis.

Why Do You Need Renal Diet?

Renal typically based on certain foods that are low in sodium, potassium, and phosphorus, which are minerals that are known to help build up fluid in the system. When you have renal disease though, these fluids cannot be easily expelled by your kidneys through the urine and so you must limit their consumption so that there is no risk of fluid build-up and worsening of the disease.

Renal diet, in general decreases the likelihood of renal disorder progression through the following ways:

- Minimizes risky fluid buildup from high levels of minerals, as the kidneys cannot process excessive amounts on their own.

- Encourages the consumption of high-quality protein, while limiting the amount of bad protein that could be damaging to the kidneys.

- Helps keep the minerals, electrolytes, and salts in our system balanced partially replacing your kidneys' function when they can't fully work on their own.

A renal diet is especially useful during stages 1-3 as it is mainly used as a preventive measure rather than an actual treatment for patients in more advanced renal disease stages. However, if you follow the diet and a healthy lifestyle, there is a very high chance to avoid dialysis and live a quality life.

The Explanation of Key Diet Words

When following a renal diet, certain nutrients are very important as they can actually make worse or improve chronic kidney disorder. Here is a brief list of the most important ones

Potassium.

Potassium is a naturally occurring mineral found in nearly all foods, in varying amounts. Our bodies need an amount of potassium to help with muscle activity as well as electrolyte balance and regulation of blood pressure. However, when there is an excessive amount of potassium in the system and the kidneys can't expel it (due to renal disease), fluid retention and muscle spasms can occur.

Phosphorus.

Phosphorus is a trace mineral found in a wide range of foods and especially dairy, meat, and eggs. It acts synergistically with calcium as well as Vitamin D to promote bone health. However, when there is damage to the kidneys, excess amounts of the mineral cannot be taken out and this can cause bone weakness.

Calories.

When being on a renal diet, it is important to give yourself the right amount of calories to fuel your system. The exact amount of calories you should consume daily depends on your age, gender, general health status, and stage of renal disease. In most cases though, there are no strict limitations in the calorie intake, as long as you take them from proper sources that are low in sodium, potassium, and phosphorus. In general, doctors recommend a daily limit between 1800-2100 calories per day to keep weight within the normal range.

Protein.

Protein is an essential nutrient that our systems need to develop and generate new connective tissue e.g. muscles, even during injuries. Protein also helps stop bleeding and helps the immune system fight infections. A healthy adult with no kidney disease would normally need 40-65 grams of protein per day.

However, in a renal diet, protein consumption is a tricky subject as too much or too little can cause problems. Protein, when being metabolized by our systems also creates waste which is typically processed by the kidneys. But when kidneys are damaged or underperforming, as in the case of kidney disease that waste will stay in the system. This is why patients in more advanced CKD stages, are advised to limit their protein consumption as well.

Fats.

Fats and particularly good fats are needed by our systems as a fuel source and for other metabolic cell functions. A diet rich in bad and trans or saturated fats though can greatly raise the odds of developing heart problems, which often occur with renal disease. This is why most physicians advise their renal patients to follow a diet that contains a decent amount of good fats and a very low amount of trans (processed) or saturated fat.

Sodium.

Sodium is an essential mineral that our bodies need to regulate fluid and electrolyte balance. It also plays a role in normal cell division in the muscles and nervous system. However, in kidney disease, sodium can quickly spike at higher than normal levels and the kidneys will be unable to expel it causing fluid accumulation as a side-effect. Those who also suffer from heart problems as well should limit its consumption as it may raise blood pressure.

Carbohydrates.

Carbs act as a major and quick fuel source for the body's cells. When we consume carbs, our systems turn them into glucose and then into energy for "feeding" our body cells. Carbs are generally not restricted in the renal diet but some types of carbs contain dietary fiber as well, which helps regulate normal colon function and protect blood vessels from damage.

Dietary Fiber.

Fiber is an important element in our system that cannot be properly digested but plays a key role in the regulation of our bowel movements and blood cell protection. The fiber in the renal diet is generally encouraged as it helps loosen up the stools, relieve constipation and bloating and protect from colon damage. However, many patients don't get enough amounts of dietary fiber per day as many of them are high in potassium or phosphorus. Fortunately, there are some good dietary fiber sources for CKD patients that have lower amounts of these minerals compared to others.

Vitamins/Minerals.

Our systems, according to medical research, need at least 13 vitamins and minerals to keep our cells fully active and healthy. Patients with renal disease though are more likely to be depleted by water-soluble vitamins like B-complex and Vitamin C, as a result, or limited fluid consumption. Therefore, supplementation with these vitamins along with a renal diet program should help cover any possible vitamin deficiencies. Supplementation of fat-soluble vitamins like vitamins A, K, and E may be avoided as they can quickly build up in the system and turn toxic.

Fluids.

When you are in an advanced stage of renal disease, fluid can quickly build-up and lead to problems. While it is important to keep your system well hydrated, you should avoid minerals like potassium and sodium which can trigger further fluid build-up and cause a host of other symptoms.

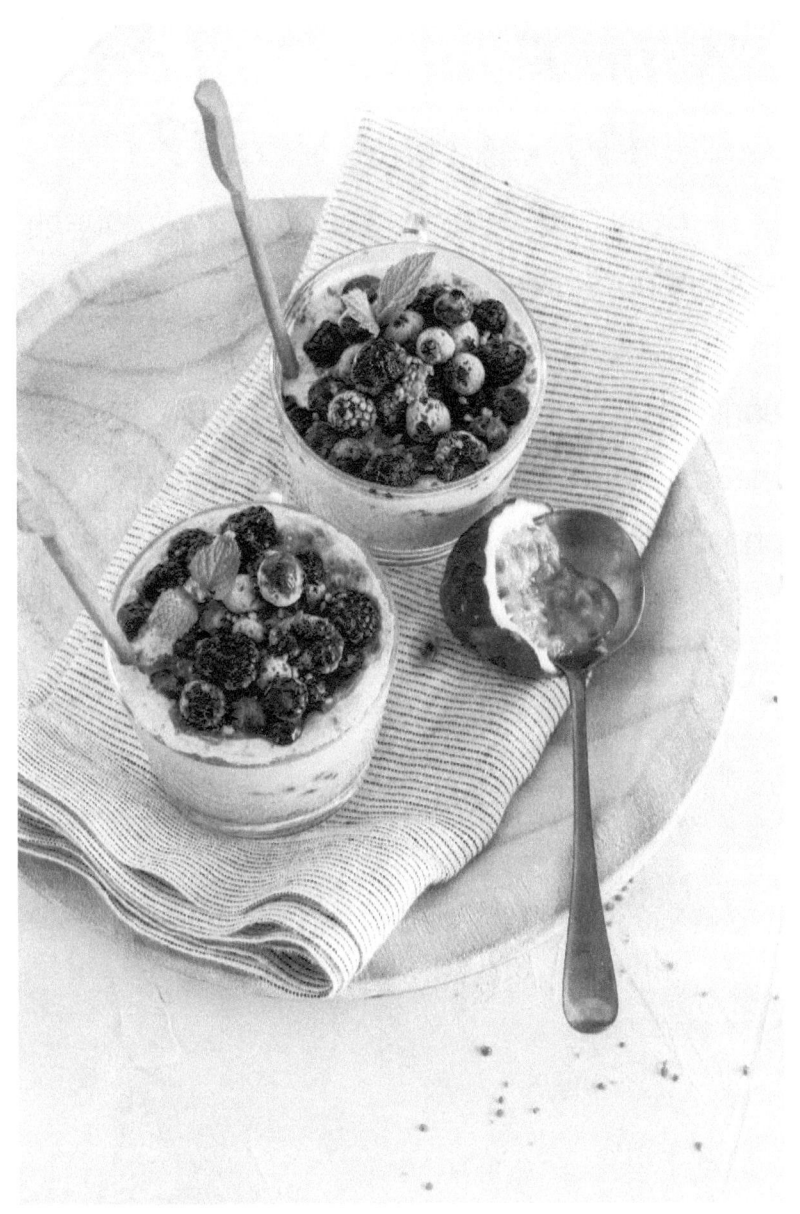

What Food to Eat and What to Avoid?

Being on a renal diet, you are probably wondering which foods you can consume and which you can avoid. As it was specified earlier, you need to consume foods that are naturally low in sodium, potassium, and phosphorus. These foods are:

- Red forest fruits e.g. berries, blueberries, strawberries, raspberries
- Red bell peppers
- Corn
- Cabbage
- Lettuce
- Broccoli
- Cauliflower
- Garlic
- Onions
- Celery
- Apples
- Cherries

- Red Grapes
- Peaches
- Figs
- Egg whites
- Vegetable oils e.g. olive oil or safflower oil
- Soy milk
- Egg whites
- Cream cheese
- Cottage cheese
- Parmesan cheese
- Fresh fish and seafood e.g. mahi-mahi tuna, lobster, crab, oysters, and shrimp
- Imitation fish e.g. crab sticks
- Pasta
- Bread
- Unfortified rice milk
- Corn cereals
- Green beans
- Radishes
- Beef (in moderate amounts)
- Turkey

- Chicken

Make sure that you eat fresh and unprocessed versions of the above as dried fruits or canned fish and meat may be possibly loaded with hidden amounts of extra sodium and phosphorus.

Now, when it comes to foods that you should avoid, although you don't have to avoid them completely for long periods, it's best to limit their consumption as they contain high amounts of sodium, phosphorus, and/or potassium:

- Avocadoes
- Bananas
- Lentils
- Beans
- Spinach
- Swiss chard
- Mature cheeses e.g. cheddar or gouda
- Cow milk
- Most dairy products

- Liver and organ meats
- Brewer's yeast
- Egg yolks
- Chocolate
- Cola's
- Custard
- Dairy ice-cream
- Potatoes
- Oranges
- Apricots
- Dried fruit
- Pickles and relish
- Packaged crisps and crackers
- Brown rice
- Most packed and canned food e.g. cream soups or spam.

Be extra cautious as phosphorus can cleverly hide in many packed food labels, under different chemical names such as:

- Phosphoric acid
- Disodium phosphate

- Monosodium phosphate
- Trisodium phosphate
- Dicalcium phosphate
- Tetrasodium pyrophosphate

If you notice any of the above names in the top 5 ingredients of a food label, it typically means that the food is high in phosphorus and should be avoided.

List of Juices and Drinks in Renal Diet

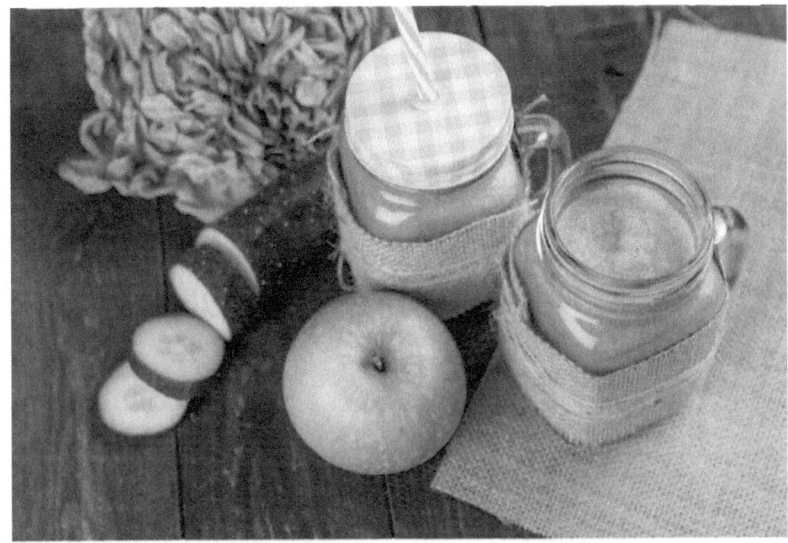

When following a renal diet, keeping yourself hydrated without exceeding the liquid limit of 2.5 liters per day is very important. If you are currently at a more progressed stage e.g. stage 4, your doctor may suggest you limit the consumption of fluids up to 2 liters per day. In most cases, you can drink:

- Plain or fruit-infused water
- Homemade ice tea
- Grape juice

- Berry juice
- Peach juice
- Green tea
- Caffeine-free herbal tea e.g. chamomile.
- Almond milk
- Soda water
- Lemonade
- Light-colored fizzy drinks e.g. sprite
- Coffee in moderate amounts
- Coffee alternatives with fig and chicory wood.
- Low-fat goat milk
- Smoothies with berries, peaches, apples, or celery blended with water or almond milk.

You may also consume low alcoholic drinks like wine and beer in moderate amounts and preferably not more than 5 cups per week.

Frequently Asked Questions

Q: How can I figure out if a food label or recipe is low in potassium and what is the maximum daily limit?

A: When following a renal diet, you ideally want to make sure that potassium levels are below 250mg/per serving or up to 7% of the food's total nutritional value. If the food/recipe indicates less than 100 mg of potassium per serving, this means that it's very low in potassium, however, a moderate rate of up to 250 mg per serving is fine, as long as you don't consume any other foods throughout the day with moderate or high potassium levels e.g. between 250-400 mg/serving.

Q: Is it possible to lose weight during a renal diet?

A: If you wish to lose extra weight for health or fitness reasons, you can follow a renal diet plan that is preferably high in fats and fiber foods e.g. forest fruits, cabbage, etc. You still want to make sure that your daily calorie intake does not exceed 2000 calories and any foods that you choose are low in sodium and potassium to keep bloating and fluid build-up under control. The exact amount of calories that you need to take though, depends on your age, gender, health status, and the weight goal that you wish to achieve. If you wish to lose weight as well with your renal diet plan, it's better to discuss the matter with an expert dietician or nutritionist.

Q: Does my CKD stage count when following a renal diet?

A: Absolutely! In earlier stages (up to the third stage), it is fine to consume low to moderate amounts of sodium, potassium, and phosphorus while your fluid intake should be up to 2.5 liters per day. However, when you are in a more advanced stage of renal damage, you have to limit all the above minerals and fluids further e.g. drink up to 2 liters of fluids per day or only up to 150 mg of potassium per meal (instead of 250mg). Your doctor or dietician will give you additional guidelines on the exact amounts of each that you need to take daily, based on your current stage of renal disease.

Q: Is it OK to take caffeine in a renal diet?

A: In most cases and especially during the first three stages of CKD, a caffeine-based drink is perfectly fine. You may drink up to 2 cups of coffee or caffeine tea per day without any worries. However, be careful as any extras that you add to your coffee will not only increase calories, they may raise potassium levels as well. Such toppings are whipping cream, caramel syrups, chocolate, etc. Pure coffee or black tea with water and a bit of almond or soy milk isn't an issue but anything "fortified" should be avoided.

Q: Can I take over the counter medication when on a renal diet?

A: Unfortunately, the vast majority of over the counter medication/painkillers like aspirin and ibuprofen are not indicated for CKD patients. Any drug that belongs in the NSAID (nonsteroidal anti-inflammatory drugs) category should be avoided as according to some studies, NSAIDs can worsen CKD. Some other types of medication are also not indicated for renal patients. If you are currently taking any other medication, it would be wise to consult your doctor to find out whether they are OK for kidney function or not.

Recipes

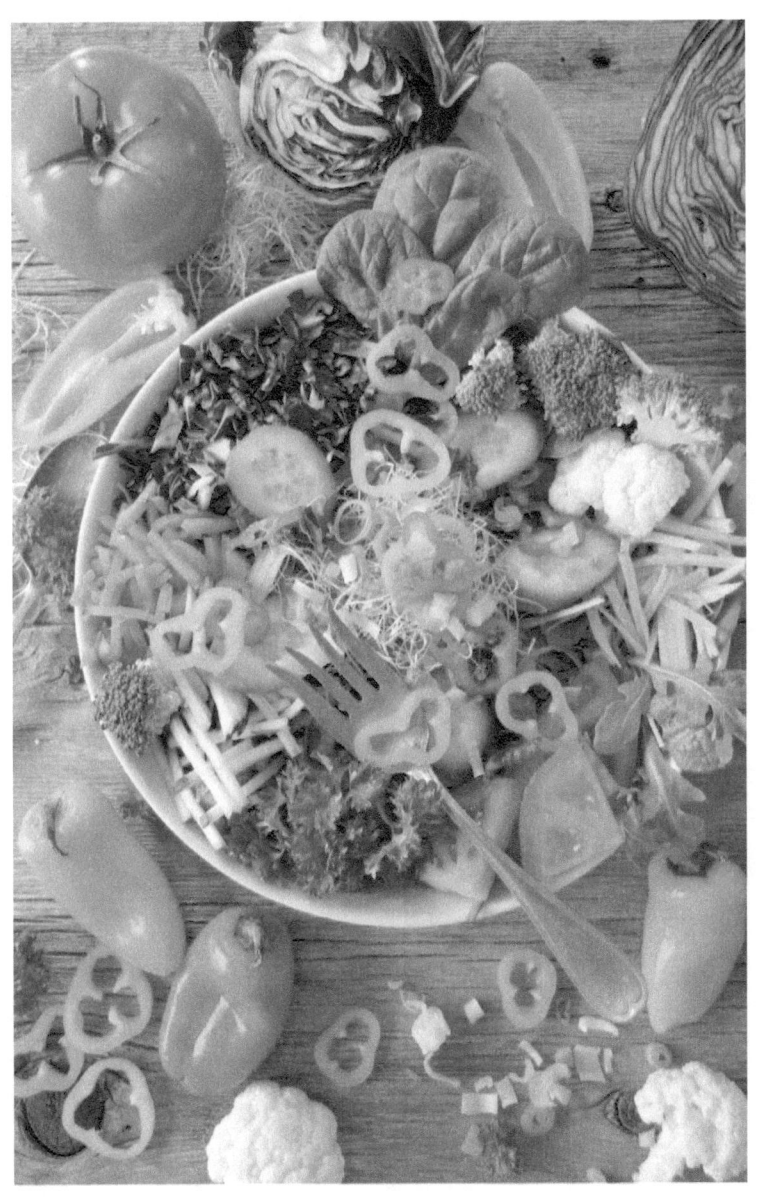

Breakfast

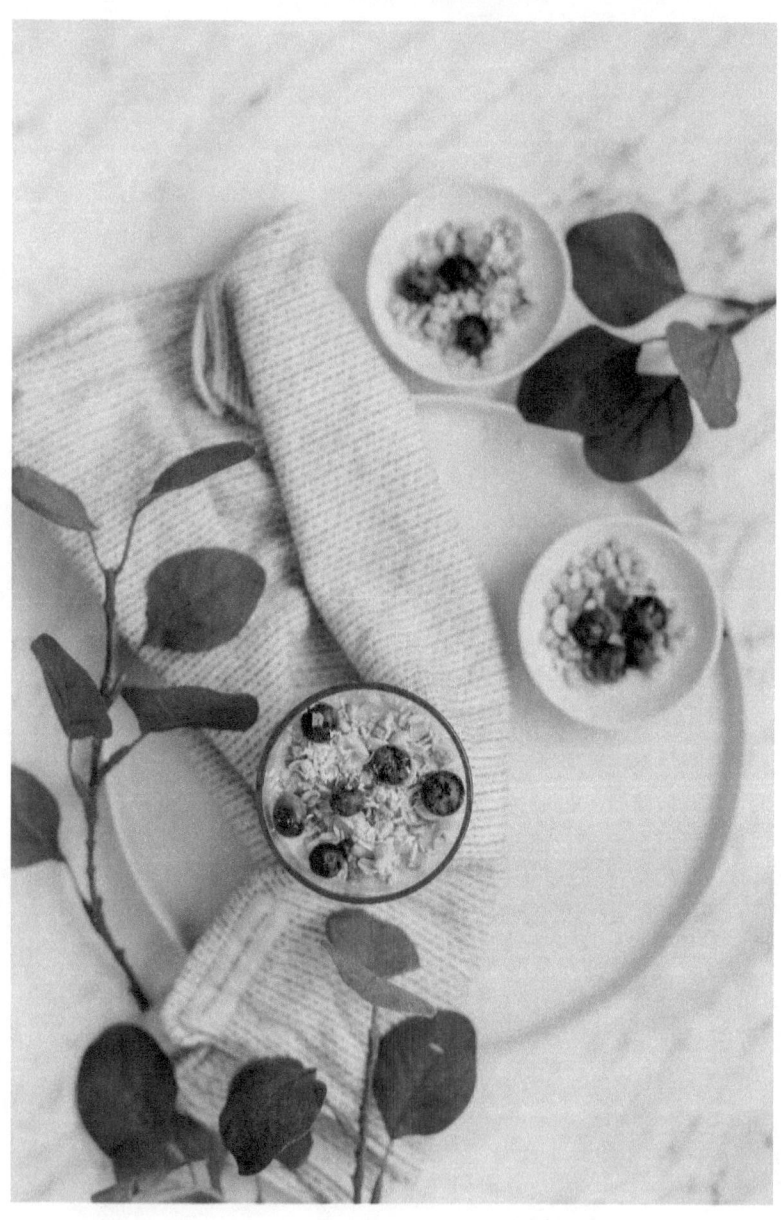

Egg White and Pepper Omelette

COOKING TIME: 5 MIN

DESCRIPTION

A low-calorie omelet recipe with red bell peppers that you can make in under 5 minutes with just 5 ingredients. Feel free to enhance its taste with paprika or Mexican spices.

INGREDIENTS FOR 1-2 SERVINGS

- 4 egg whites, lightly beaten
- 1 red bell pepper, diced
- 1 tsp of paprika
- 2 tbsp of olive oil
- ½ tsp of salt
- Pepper

METHOD

1. In a shallow pan (around 8 inches), heat the olive oil and saute the bell peppers until softened.
2. Add the egg whites and the paprika and fold the edges into the fluid center with a spatula and let the omelet cook until eggs are fully opaque and solid.
3. Season with salt and pepper.
4. Serve.

NUTRITIONAL INFORMATION (Per Serving)

- Calories: 165 kcal
- Carbohydrate: 3.8 g
- Protein: 9.2 g
- Sodium: 797 mg
- Potassium: 193 mg
- Phosphorus: 202.5 mg
- Dietary Fiber: 0.7 g
- Fat: 15.22 g
- Sugar: 0 g

Blueberry Smoothie Bowl

COOKING TIME: 1 MIN

DESCRIPTION

An Instagram worthy purple smoothie bowl made with frozen blueberries that are fortified with antioxidants. Plus, it counts less than 150 mg of potassium and phosphorus per serving.

INGREDIENTS FOR 1 SERVING

- ½ cup of frozen blueberries
- ½ cup of vanilla-flavored almond milk
- 1 tbsp of agave syrup
- 1 tsp of chia seeds

METHOD

1. Combine everything except for the chia seeds in the blender until smooth. You should end up with a thick smoothie paste.

2. Transfer into a cereal bowl and top with chia seeds on top.

NUTRITIONAL INFORMATION (Per Serving)

- Calories: 278.5 kcal
- Carbohydrate: 38.72 g
- Protein: 1.3 g
- Sodium: 76.33 mg
- Potassium: 229.1 mg
- Phosphorus: 59.2 mg
- Dietary Fiber: 7.4 g
- Fat: 6 g
- Sugar: 14 g

Turkey Breakfast Sausage

COOKING TIME: 6 MIN

DESCRIPTION

Fancy a quick sausage for breakfast or brunch? Try this low potassium breakfast sausage with turkey and spices-feel free to serve this with cornbread and apple sauce.

INGREDIENTS FOR 12 SERVINGS (12 patties per recipe)

- 1 pound of lean ground turkey
- 1 tsp of fennel seed
- ¼ tsp garlic powder
- ¼ tsp onion powder
- ¼ tsp salt
- 2 tbsp of vegetable oil
- Pepper

METHOD

1. Combine all the ingredients apart from the vegetable oil in a mixing bowl.
2. Form into long and flat (around 4 inch-long) patties.
3. Heat the vegetable oil in a medium frying pan.
4. Add 3-4 patties at a time and cook for approx. 3 minutes on each side. Repeat until you cook all the patties.
5. Serve warm.

NUTRITIONAL INFORMATION (Per Serving)

- Calories: 74 kcal
- Carbohydrate: 0.1 g
- Protein: 7 g
- Sodium: 121.9 mg
- Potassium: 89.5 mg
- Phosphorus: 75 mg
- Dietary Fiber: 0 g
- Fat: 5.16 g
- Sugar: 0.03 g

Italian Apple Fritters

COOKING TIME: 8 MIN

DESCRIPTION

A quick apple fritter recipe with cornflour batter that is great for breakfast and dessert too. Make this preferably in a deep fryer and enjoy hot as it will lose its crisp after a few minutes.

INGREDIENTS FOR 4 SERVINGS

- 2 large apples, seeded, peeled, and thickly sliced in circles
- 3 tbsp of cornflour
- ½ tsp of water
- 1 tsp of sugar
- 1 tsp of cinnamon
- Vegetable oil (for frying)
- Sprinkle of icing sugar or honey

METHOD

1. In a small bowl, combine the cornflour, water, and sugar to make your batter

2. Deep the apple rounds into the cornflour mix.
3. Heat enough vegetable oil to cover half of the pan's surface over medium to high heat.
4. Add the apple rounds into the pan and cook until golden brown.
5. Transfer into a shallow dish with absorbing paper on top and sprinkle with a bit of cinnamon and icing sugar.

NUTRITIONAL INFORMATION (Per Serving)

- Calories: 183 kcal
- Carbohydrate: 17.9 g
- Protein: 0.3 g
- Sodium: 2 g
- Potassium: 100 mg
- Phosphorus: 12.5 mg
- Dietary Fiber: 1.4 g
- Fat: 14.17 g
- Sugar: 9.3 g

Tofu and Mushroom Scramble

COOKING TIME: 7-8 MIN

DESCRIPTION

A hearty mushroom scramble recipe for vegans or fans of earthy mushroom flavors enhanced by a fine blend of exotic spices. Great for breakfast or a delicious savory brunch.

INGREDIENTS FOR 2 SERVINGS

- ½ cup of sliced white mushrooms
- ⅓ cup medium-firm tofu, crumbled
- 1 tbsp of chopped shallots
- ⅓ tsp turmeric
- 1 tsp of cumin
- ⅓ tsp of smoked paprika
- ½ tsp of garlic salt
- Pepper
- 3 tbsp of vegetable oil

METHOD

1. Heat the oil in a medium frying pan and saute the sliced mushrooms with the shallots until softened (around 3-4 minutes) over medium to high heat.
2. Add the tofu pieces and toss in the spices and the garlic salt. Toss lightly until tofu and mushrooms are nicely combined.
3. Serve warm.

NUTRITIONAL INFORMATION (Per Serving)

- Calories: 220 kcal
- Carbohydrate: 2.59 g
- Protein: 3.2 g
- Sodium: 288 mg
- Potassium: 133.5 mg
- Phosphorus: 68.5 mg
- Dietary Fiber: 1.7 g
- Fat: 23.7 g
- Sugar: 5 g

Sunny Pineapple Breakfast Smoothie

COOKING TIME: 1 MIN

DESCRIPTION

A sunny and bright breakfast smoothie with the sweet and sour goodness of pineapple blended with a hint of ginger for that zingy fresh taste.

INGREDIENTS FOR 1 SERVING.

- ½ cup of frozen pineapple chunks
- ⅔ cup almond milk
- ½ tsp of ginger powder
- 1 tbsp of agave syrup

METHOD

1. Blend everything in a blender until nice and smooth (around 30 seconds).
2. Transfer into a tall glass or mason jar.
3. Serve and enjoy.

NUTRITIONAL INFORMATION (Per Serving)

- Calories: 186 kcal
- Carbohydrate: 43.7 g
- Protein: 2.28 g
- Sodium: 130 mg
- Potassium: 135 mg
- Phosphorus: 18 mg
- Dietary Fiber: 2.4 g
- Fat: 2.3 g
- Sugar: 17.2 g

Puff Oven Pancakes

COOKING TIME: 30 MIN

DESCRIPTION

A crunchy oven pancake recipe with rice flour that is very low in potassium and phosphorus. Try this if you want something crunchy and interesting compared to ordinary pancakes.

INGREDIENTS FOR 4 SERVINGS

- 2 large eggs.
- ½ cup of rice flour
- ½ cup of rice milk
- 2 tbsp of unsalted butter
- ⅛ tsp salt

METHOD

1. Preheat the oven at 400F/190C.
2. Grease a 10-inch skillet or Pyrex with the butter and heat in the oven until it melts.

3. In a mixing bowl, beat the eggs and whisk in the rice milk, flour and salt until smooth.
4. Take off the skillet or pie dish from the oven.
5. Transfer directly the batter into the skillet and put back in the oven for 25-30 minutes.
6. Place in a serving dish and cut into 4 portions.
7. Serve hot with honey or icing sugar on top.

NUTRITIONAL INFORMATION (Per Serving)
- Calories: 159.75 kcal
- Carbohydrate: 17 g
- Protein: 5 g
- Sodium: 120 g
- Potassium: 52 mg
- Phosphorus: 66.25 mg
- Dietary Fiber: 0.5 g
- Fat: 9 g

- Sugar: 1.6 g

Savory Muffins with Protein

COOKING TIME 35 MIN

DESCRIPTION

A great alternative to sweet and tangy blueberry muffins. This savory muffin recipe is great alone or as a part of your breakfast. You can take it with some bacon or homemade sausage on the side and it will be delicious.

INGREDIENTS FOR 12 SERVINGS

- 2 cups of corn flakes
- ½ cup of unfortified almond milk
- 4 large eggs
- 2 tbsp of olive oil
- 1/2 cup of almond milk
- 1 medium white onion, sliced
- 1 cup of plain Greek yogurt
- ¼ cup pecans, chopped
- 1 tbsp of mixed seasoning blend e.g. Mrs. dash

METHOD
1. Preheat the oven at 350F/180C.
2. Heat the olive oil in the pan. Saute the onions with the pecans and seasoning blend for a couple of minutes.
3. Add the rest of the ingredients and toss well.
4. Split the mixture into 12 small muffin cups (lightly greased) and bake for 30-35 minutes or until an inserted knife or toothpick is coming out clean.
5. Serve warm or keep at room temperature for a couple of days.

NUTRITIONAL INFORMATION (Per Serving)

- Calories: 106.58 kcal
- Carbohydrate: 8.20 g
- Protein: 4.77 g
- Sodium: 51.91 mg
- Potassium: 87.83 mg
- Phosphorus: 49.41 mg
- Dietary Fiber: 0.58 g

- Fat: 5 g
- Sugar: 1.23 g

Tex-Mex Sausage

COOKING TIME: 12 MIN

DESCRIPTION

Delicious Tex-Mex sausage recipe that is spicy and hearty enough for a weekend's lazy brunch. The combo of spices and flavors really makes up for the low amount of sodium.

INGREDIENTS FOR 8 SERVINGS

- ½ pound of lean ground beef
- ¼ cup of white onion, thinly chopped
- 1 large clove of garlic, minced
- 1 tbsp of fresh cilantro, chopped
- 1 tbsp of vinegar
- 2 tbsp of canned green chili peppers
- ¼ tsp salt
- 1 tsp of chili powder

METHOD

1. In a mixing bowl, mix cilantro, onions, green chili peppers, garlic, vinegar, and chili powder.
2. Add the ground beef and mix again everything well.
3. Form the mixture into 8 equal flat or semi-flat patties.
4. Grease a skillet with a bit of vegetable oil. Place the patties on the pan over medium heat and let cook for 5-6 minutes on each side.

NUTRITIONAL INFORMATION (Per Serving)

- Calories: 88 kcal
- Carbohydrate: 1 g
- Protein: 11.58 g
- Sodium: 80 mg
- Potassium: 105 mg
- Phosphorus: 64 mg
- Dietary Fiber: 0.4 g
- Fat: 9 g
- Sugar: 0.5 g

European Pancakes

COOKING TIME: 15-20 MIN

DESCRIPTION

European pancakes, most favored by the French and the Germans are thin and soft and make an excellent base for other dishes-both savory and sweet. If you are making these for breakfast, top them with some fresh strawberries and honey for a low potassium sweet treat.

INGREDIENTS FOR 10 SERVINGS (20 pancakes)

- 2/3 cups of all-purpose flour
- 4 large eggs
- 2 tbsp of sugar
- ½ tsp of lemon zest
- 1 cup of low-fat milk
- ¼ tsp of vanilla extract

METHOD

1. In a medium bowl, mix the flour with the sugar. Whisk in the eggs and combine well.
2. Add the milk, vanilla, and lemon zest to the mix and whisk well.
3. Spray a small 8-10 inch pan with cooking spray and pour around 4 tbsp of the mixture and distribute evenly by tilting the pan from one side to another.
4. Cook until the batter is solid and light golden brown (around 50 seconds on each side). Flip.
5. Repeat the above two steps until all the batter has finished.
6. Serve.

NUTRITIONAL INFORMATION (Per Serving)

- Calories: 74 kcal
- Carbohydrate: 10 g
- Protein: 4 g
- Sodium: 39 mg
- Potassium: 73 mg

- Phosphorus: 73 mg
- Dietary Fiber: 0.2 g
- Fat: 2 g
- Sugar: 1.2 g

Multigrain Warm Porridge

COOKING TIME: 30 MIN

DESCRIPTION

A hearty breakfast recipe that combines 3 types of low potassium grains along with oats for a nice contrast of flavors and textures. If you have 30 minutes to spare, you need to try this.

INGREDIENTS FOR 2 SERVINGS

- 2 cups of water
- 2 tbsp of old fashioned grits
- 1 tbsp of uncooked roasted buckwheat
- 1 tbsp of steel-cut oats, uncooked
- 3 tbsp of plain couscous
- 1 tsp of honey
- 1 tsp of cinnamon

METHOD

1. Bring the water to boil in a small pot.
2. Add grits and stir for a few seconds.

3. Add the buckwheat and the oats, stir for a few seconds and lower the heat. Cover the pot and let simmer for 20 minutes.
4. Remove the lid from the pot and add the couscous. Take off the heat and let sit covered for another 5 minutes.
5. Transfer into a cereal bowl and sprinkle some honey and cinnamon or blueberries on top.

NUTRITIONAL INFORMATION (Per Serving)

- Calories: 298 kcal
- Carbohydrate: 60.3 g
- Protein: 9 g
- Sodium: 0.5 g
- Potassium: 78 mg
- Phosphorus: 25.2 mg
- Dietary Fiber: 3 g
- Fat: 1 g
- Sugar: 0 g

Puffy French Toast

COOKING TIME: 8 MIN

DESCRIPTION

An easy French toast recipe that is dairy-free for lower amounts of phosphorus. Made in the pan and finished in the oven for an extra puffy result.

INGREDIENTS FOR 4 SERVINGS

- 4 slices of white bread, cut in half diagonally
- 3 whole eggs and 1 egg white
- 1 cup of plain almond milk
- 2 tbsp of canola oil
- 1 tsp of cinnamon

METHOD

1. Preheat your oven to 400F/180C
2. Beat together the eggs with the almond milk.
3. Heat the oil in a pan.

4. Dip each bread slice/triangle into the egg and almond milk mixture.
5. Fry in the pan until golden brown on each side.
6. Place the toasts in a baking dish and let cook in the oven for another 5 minutes.
7. Serve warm and drizzle with some honey, icing sugar, or cinnamon on top.

NUTRITIONAL INFORMATION (Per Serving)

- Calories: 293.75 kcal
- Carbohydrate: 25.3 g
- Protein: 9.27 g
- Sodium: 211 g
- Potassium: 97 mg
- Phosphorus: 165 mg
- Dietary Fiber: 12.3 g
- Fat: 16.50 g
- Sugar: 1.6 g

Lunch

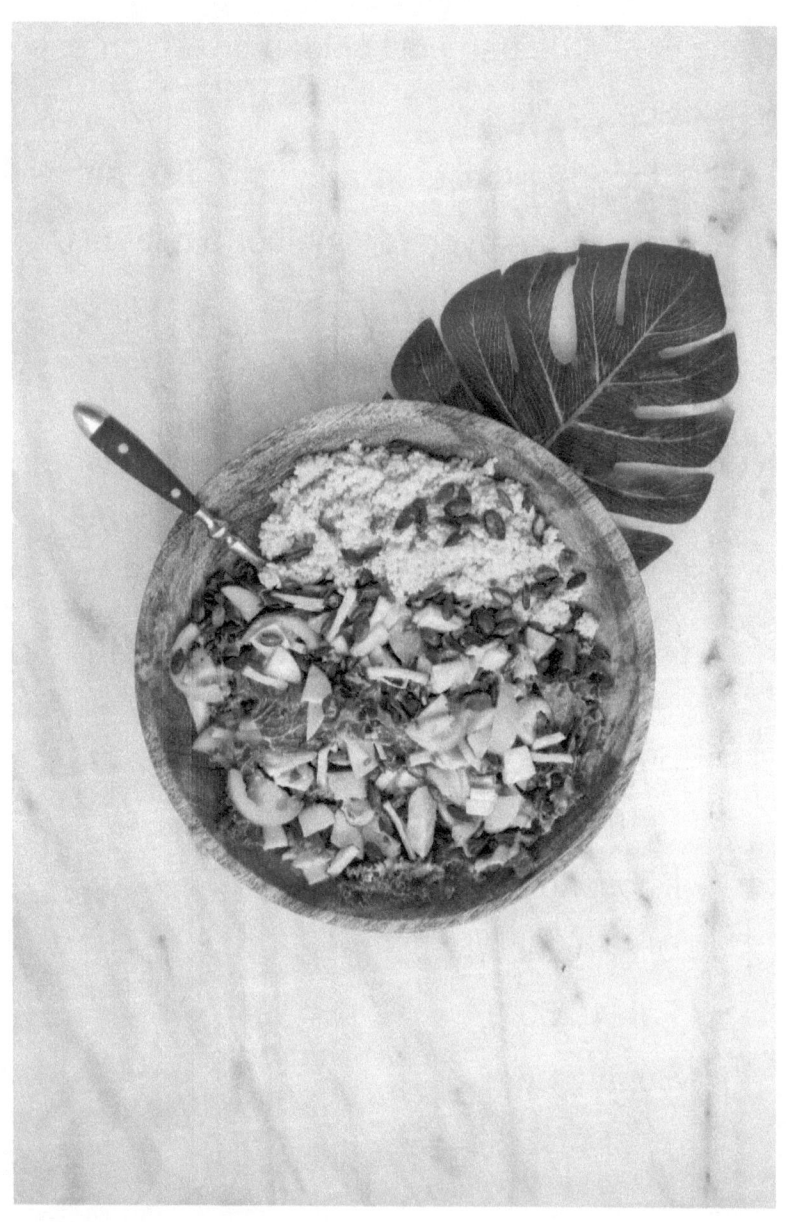

Couscous with Veggies

COOKING TIME: 10 MIN

DESCRIPTION

Couscous is my favorite grain as it's very easy and quick to make. If you wish to have your daily dose of veggies in a more delicious and easy to eat way, try this recipe.

INGREDIENTS FOR 5 SERVINGS

- ½ cup of uncooked couscous
- ¼ cup of white mushrooms, sliced
- ½ cup of red onion, chopped
- 1 garlic clove, minced
- ½ cup of frozen peas
- 2 tbsp of dry white wine
- ½ tsp of basil
- 2 tbsp of fresh parsley, chopped
- 1 cup water or vegetable stock
- 1 tbsp of margarine or vegetable oil

METHOD

1. Thaw the peas by setting them aside at room temperature for 15-20 minutes.
2. In a medium pan, heat the margarine or vegetable oil.
3. Add the onions, peas, mushroom, and garlic and saute for around 5 minutes. Add the wine and let it evaporate.
4. Add all the herbs and spices and toss well. Take off the heat and keep aside.
5. In a small pot, cook the couscous with 1 cup of hot water or vegetable stock. Bring to a boil, take off the heat and let sit for a few minutes with a lid covered.
6. Add the saute veggies to the couscous and toss well.
7. Serve in a serving bowl warm or cold.

NUTRITIONAL INFORMATION (Per Serving)

- Calories: 110.4 kcal
- Carbohydrate: 18 g
- Protein: 3 g
- Sodium: 112.2 mg

- Potassium: 69.6 mg
- Phosphorus: 46.8 mg
- Dietary Fiber: 2.1 g
- Fat: 2 g
- Sugar: 3.36 g

Mexican Steak Tacos

COOKING TIME: 15 MIN

DESCRIPTION

Tacos are a trademark dish of Mexican cuisine and if you wish to make them like Tex-Mex, here is a taco recipe with steak as the key ingredient.

INGREDIENTS FOR 8 SERVINGS.

- 1 pound of flank or skirt steak
- ¼ cup of fresh cilantro, chopped
- ¼ cup white onion, chopped
- 3 limes, juiced
- 3 cloves of garlic, minced
- 2 tsp of garlic powder
- 2 tbsp of olive oil
- ½ cup of Mexican or mozzarella cheese, grated
- 1 tsp of Mexican seasoning
- 8 medium-sized (6") corn flour tortillas.

METHOD

1. Combine the juice from two limes, Mexican seasoning, and garlic powder in a dish or bowl and marinate the steak with it for at least half an hour in the fridge.
2. In a separate bowl, combine the chopped cilantro, garlic, onion, and juice from one lime to make your salsa. Cover and keep in the fridge.
3. Heat the olive oil in a medium pan. Slice steak into thin strips and cook for approx. 3 minutes on each side.
4. Preheat your oven to 350F/180C.
5. Distribute evenly the steak strips in each tortilla. Top with a tablespoon of the grated cheese on top.
6. Wrap each taco in aluminum foil and bake in the oven for approx. 7-8 minutes or until cheese is melted.
7. Serve warm with your cilantro salsa.

NUTRITIONAL INFORMATION (Per Serving)

- Calories: 230 kcal
- Carbohydrate: 19.5 g
- Protein: 15 g
- Sodium: 486.75 g
- Potassium: 240 mg
- Phosphorus: 268 mg
- Dietary Fiber: 0.1 g
- Fat: 11 g
- Sugar: 1.2 g

Beer Pork Ribs

COOKING TIME: 8 HOURS

DESCRIPTION

A juicy pork ribs recipe made with root beer and three other ingredients for minimal fuss. If you have a slow cooker and wish to have a delicious family meal for lunch, this is worth trying out.

INGREDIENTS FOR 6 SERVINGS.

- 2 pounds of pork ribs, cut in two units/racks
- 18 oz. of root beer
- 2 cloves of garlic, minced
- 2 tbsp of onion powder
- 2 tbsp of vegetable oil (optional)

METHOD

1. Wrap the pork ribs with vegetable oil and place one unit on the bottom of your slow

cooker with half of the minced garlic and the onion powder. Place the other rack on top with the rest of the garlic and onion powder.
2. Pour over the root beer and cover the lid.
3. Let simmer for 8 hours on low heat.
4. Take off and finish optionally in a grilling pan for a nice sear.

NUTRITIONAL INFORMATION (Per Serving)

- Calories: 301 kcal
- Carbohydrate: 36 g
- Protein: 21 g
- Sodium: 729 mg
- Potassium: 200 mg
- Phosphorus: 209 mg
- Dietary Fiber: 0 g
- Fat: 18 g
- Sugar: 10 g

Crispy Lemon Chicken

COOKING TIME: 10 MIN

DESCRIPTION

This delicious lemon chicken recipe looks complex but it's actually very easy to cook. The breading also adds a nice crunch to its lemony sauce.

INGREDIENTS FOR 6 SERVINGS

- 1 pound of boneless and skinless, chicken breast
- ½ cup of all-purpose flour
- 1 large egg
- ½ cup of lemon juice
- 2 tbsp of water
- ¼ tsp salt
- ¼ tsp lemon pepper
- 1 tsp of mixed herb seasoning
- 2 tbsp of olive oil
- A few lemon slices for garnishing

- 1 tbsp of chopped parsley (for garnishing)
- 2 cups of cooked plain white rice

METHOD

1. Cut the chicken breast into thin slices and season with the herb seasoning, salt, and pepper.
2. In a small bowl, whisk together the egg with the water.
3. Keep the flour in a separate bowl.
4. Dip the chicken slices in the egg bath and then into the flour. Ensure that all sides are coated with flour.
5. Heat your oil in a medium frying pan.
6. Shallow fry the chicken in the pan until golden brown (approx. 3 minutes on each side).
7. Add the lemon juice and cook for another couple of minutes.
8. Taken the chicken out of the pan and transfer it to a wide dish with absorbing paper to absorb any excess oil.

9. Garnish with some chopped parsley and lemon wedges on top and serve with the cooked white rice.

NUTRITIONAL INFORMATION (Per Serving)

- Calories: 232 kcal
- Carbohydrate: 24 g
- Protein: 18 g
- Sodium: 100 g
- Potassium: 234 mg
- Phosphorus: 217 mg
- Dietary Fiber: 0.8 g
- Fat: 8 g
- Sugar: 0.3 g

Mexican Chorizo Sausage

COOKING TIME: 15 MIN

DESCRIPTION

A sausage patty enhanced with true Mexican and Spanish flavors that fans of mildly spicy food will love. Serve ideally with Mexican salsa and some roasted veggies.

INGREDIENTS FOR 16 SERVINGS.

- 2 pounds of boneless pork but, coarsely ground
- 3 tbsp of red wine vinegar
- 2 tbsp of smoked paprika
- ½ tsp of cinnamon
- ½ tsp of ground cloves
- ¼ tsp of coriander seeds
- ¼ tsp ground ginger
- 1 tsp of ground cumin
- 3 tbsp of brandy

METHOD

1. In a large mixing bowl, combine the ground pork with the seasonings, brandy, and vinegar and mix with your hands well.
2. Place the mixture into a large Ziploc bag and leave it in the fridge overnight, for all the flavors to blend and for lightly curing the sausage.
3. Form into 15-16 patties of equal size.
4. Heat the oil in a large pan and fry the patties for approx. 5-7 minutes on each side, or until the meat inside is no longer pink and there is a light brown crust on top.
5. Serve hot.

NUTRITIONAL INFORMATION (Per Serving)

- Calories: 134 kcal
- Carbohydrate: 0 g
- Protein: 10 g
- Sodium: 40 mg
- Potassium: 138 mg

- Phosphorus: 128 mg
- Dietary Fiber: 0 g
- Fat: 7 g
- Sugar: 0 g

Eggplant Casserole

COOKING TIME: 25-30 MIN

DESCRIPTION

Eggplant is one of these veggies that people either love or hate, but if you cook it along with other ingredients, as in this casserole recipe it makes an incredibly delicious meal for the entire family.

INGREDIENTS FOR 4 SERVINGS.

- 3 cups of eggplant, peeled and cut into large chunks
- 2 egg whites
- 1 large egg, whole
- ½ cup of unsweetened vegetable e.g. soy or almond cream
- ¼ tsp of sage
- ½ cup of breadcrumbs
- 1 tbsp of margarine, melted
- 1/4 tsp garlic salt

METHOD

1. Preheat the oven at 350F/180C.
2. Place the eggplants chunks in a medium pan, cover with a bit of water and let cook with the lid covered until tender. Drain from the water and mash with a tool or fork.
3. Beat the eggs with the non-dairy vegetable cream, sage, salt, and pepper. Whisk in the eggplant mush.
4. Combine the melted margarine with the breadcrumbs.
5. Bake in the oven for 20-25 minutes or until the casserole has a golden-brown crust.

NUTRITIONAL INFORMATION (Per Serving)

- Calories: 186 kcal
- Carbohydrate: 19 g
- Protein: 7 g
- Sodium: 503 mg

- Potassium: 230 mg
- Phosphorus: 62 mg
- Dietary Fiber: 17.4 g
- Fat: 9 g
- Sugar: 11.7 g

Easy Cilantro Cod

COOKING TIME: 8 MIN

DESCRIPTION

An incredibly easy recipe made with the fresh, sharp, and zesty flavors of lemon and cilantro. Make this with cod preferably but feel free to substitute with tilapia or haddock.

INGREDIENTS FOR 4 SERVINGS

- 1 pound of cod fillets, at room temperature
- ½ cup of mayonnaise
- ½ cup of fresh cilantro, chopped
- 2 tbsp of lime juice

METHOD

1. In a mixing bowl, mix the mayo with the cilantro and lime juice. Keep a ¼ cup in a small bowl as a sauce to serve with the cod later.

2. Brush the remaining mayo mix on the fish.
3. Heat a bit of oil in a shallow big pan over medium heat. Add the cod fillets and cook for approx. 3-4 minutes on each side.
4. Serve with the reserved cilantro and mayo sauce.

NUTRITIONAL INFORMATION (Per Serving)

- Calories: 322 kcal
- Carbohydrate: 1 g
- Protein: 26 g
- Sodium: 612 g
- Potassium: 237 mg
- Phosphorus: 218 mg
- Dietary Fiber: 0 g
- Fat: 23 g
- Sugar: 0.5 g

Light Greek Soutzoukakia

COOKING TIME: 30 MIN

DESCRIPTION

"Soutzoukakia" is a Greek/Turkish meatball that passed along many generations of Greeks and is renowned for the spicy and aromatic taste. Here is a lighter version of the original recipe.

INGREDIENTS FOR 8-10 SERVINGS

- 1 pound of ground beef (around 90% lean)
- 2 tbsp of red wine
- 1 tbsp of cumin
- 1 tsp of cinnamon
- ½ tsp of nutmeg
- ½ tsp of black pepper
- 2 tbsp of bread crumbs
- 1 large egg white
- ½ cup of tomato sauce
- Olive oil

METHOD
1. Preheat the oven at 350F/180C.
2. Mix all the ingredients in a mixing bowl.
3. Grease your hands and a baking tray with a bit of olive oil. Shape with your greased hands into small yet elongated meatballs (around 20-25 in pieces in total).
4. Bake in the oven for 30 minutes.
5. Heat the ready-made tomato sauce for 5 minutes and pour over the Soutzoukakia.

NUTRITIONAL INFORMATION (Per Serving)

- Calories: 174 kcal
- Carbohydrate: 8.1 g
- Protein: 19.8 g
- Sodium: 126 mg
- Potassium: 200 mg
- Phosphorus: 95.5 mg
- Dietary Fiber: 1.2 g
- Fat: 8.8 g
- Sugar: 0.6 g

Pizza with Chicken & Pesto

COOKING TIME: 25 MIN

DESCRIPTION

This low potassium pizza recipe is easy to make and has a burst of flavors. Try it with chicken and pesto, that blends ideally Italian and American flavors.

INGREDIENTS FOR 4 SERVINGS

- 1 ready-made frozen pizza dough
- ⅔ cup cooked chicken, chopped
- ½ cup of orange bell pepper, diced
- ½ cup of green bell pepper, diced
- ¼ cup of purple onion, chopped
- 2 tbsp of green basil pesto
- 1 tbsp of chives, chopped
- ⅓ cup of parmesan or Romano cheese, grated
- ¼ cup of mozzarella cheese
- 1 tbsp of olive oil

METHOD

1. Thaw the pizza dough according to instructions on the package.
2. Heat the olive oil in a pan and saute the peppers and onions for a couple of minutes. Set aside
3. Once the pizza dough has thawed, spread the basil pesto over its surface.
4. Top with half of the cheese, the peppers, the onions, and the chicken. Finish with the rest of the cheese.
5. Bake at 350F/180C for approx. 20 minutes (or until crust and cheese are baked).
6. Slice in triangles with a pizza cutter or sharp knife and serve.

NUTRITIONAL INFORMATION (Per Serving)

- Calories: 225 kcal
- Carbohydrate: 13.9 g
- Protein: 11.1 g

- Sodium: 321 mg
- Potassium: 174 mg
- Phosphorus: 172 mg
- Dietary Fiber: 1.2 g
- Fat: 12 g
- Sugar: 1.8 g

Easy Egg Salad

COOKING TIME: 8 MIN

DESCRIPTION

A quick and easy version of the old-school egg salad recipe that is perfect for making ahead of school or work lunch. Combine ideally in lettuce wraps or white bread as a sandwich filling.

INGREDIENTS FOR 4 SERVINGS

- 4 large eggs
- ½ cup of sweet onion, chopped
- ¼ cup of celery, chopped
- 2 tbsp of pickle relish
- 1 tbsp of yellow mustard
- 1 tsp of smoked paprika
- 3 tbsp of mayo

METHOD

1. Hard boil the eggs in a small pot filled with water for approx. 7-8 minutes. Leave

the eggs in the water for an extra couple of minutes before peeling.
2. Peel the eggs and chop finely with a knife or tool.
3. Combine all the chopped veggies with the mayo and mustard. Add in the eggs and mix well.
4. Sprinkle with some smoked paprika on top.
5. Serve cold with pitta, white bread slices, or lettuce wraps.

NUTRITIONAL INFORMATION (Per Serving)

- Calories: 127 kcal
- Carbohydrate: 6 g
- Protein: 7 g
- Sodium: 170.7 mg
- Potassium: 87.5 mg
- Phosphorus: 101 mg
- Dietary Fiber: 0.17 g
- Fat: 13 g
- Sugar: 1 g

Shrimp Quesadilla

COOKING TIME: 10 MIN

DESCRIPTION

Quesadilla is a favorite Tex-Mex lunch for kids and you can make it for lunch using two corn flour tortillas and filled with a nice blend of shrimps, peppers, and cheese inside.

INGREDIENTS FOR 2 SERVINGS

- 5 oz of shrimp, shelled and deveined
- 4 tbsp of Mexican salsa
- 2 tbsp of fresh cilantro, chopped
- 1 tbsp of lemon juice
- 1 tsp of ground cumin
- 1 tsp of cayenne pepper
- 2 tbsp of unsweetened soy yogurt or creamy tofu
- 2 medium corn flour tortillas
- 2 tbsp of low-fat cheddar cheese

METHOD

1. Mix the cilantro, cumin, lemon juice, and cayenne in a Ziploc bag to make your marinade. Add the shrimps and marinate for 10 minutes.
2. Heat a pan over medium heat with some olive oil and toss in the shrimp with the marinade. Let cook for a couple of minutes or as soon as shrimps have turned pink and opaque.
3. Add the soy cream or soft tofu to the pan and mix well. Remove from the heat and keep the marinade aside.
4. Heat tortillas in the grill or microwave for a few seconds.
5. Place 2 tbsp of salsa on each tortilla. Top one tortilla with the shrimp mixture and add the cheese on top.
6. Stack one tortilla against each other (with the spread salsa layer facing the shrimp mixture).

7. Transfer this to a baking tray and cook for 7-8 minutes at 350F/180C to melt the cheese and crisp up the tortillas.
8. Serve warm.

NUTRITIONAL INFORMATION (Per Serving)

- Calories: 255 kcal
- Carbohydrate: 21 g
- Protein: 24 g
- Sodium: 562 g
- Potassium: 235 mg
- Phosphorus: 189 mg
- Dietary Fiber: 2 g
- Fat: 9 g
- Sugar: 3 g

Grilled Corn on the Cob

COOKING TIME: 20 MIN

DESCRIPTION

A barbeque favorite for vegans and meat-eaters alike that instantly brightens your mood and satisfy your appetite.

INGREDIENTS FOR 4 SERVINGS

- 4 frozen corn on the cob, cut in half
- ½ tsp of thyme
- 1 tbsp of grated parmesan cheese
- ¼ tsp of black pepper

METHOD

1. Combine the oil, cheese, thyme, and black pepper in a bowl.
2. Place the corn in the cheese/oil mix and roll to coat evenly.
3. Fold all 4 pieces in aluminum foil, leaving a small open surface on top.

4. Place the wrapped corns over the grill and let cook for 20 minutes.
5. Serve hot.

NUTRITIONAL INFORMATION (Per Serving)

- Calories: 125 kcal
- Carbohydrate: 29.5 g
- Protein: 2 g
- Sodium: 26 g
- Potassium: 145 mg
- Phosphorus: 91.5 mg
- Dietary Fiber: 3.5 g
- Fat: 1.3 g
- Sugar: 0 g

Dinner

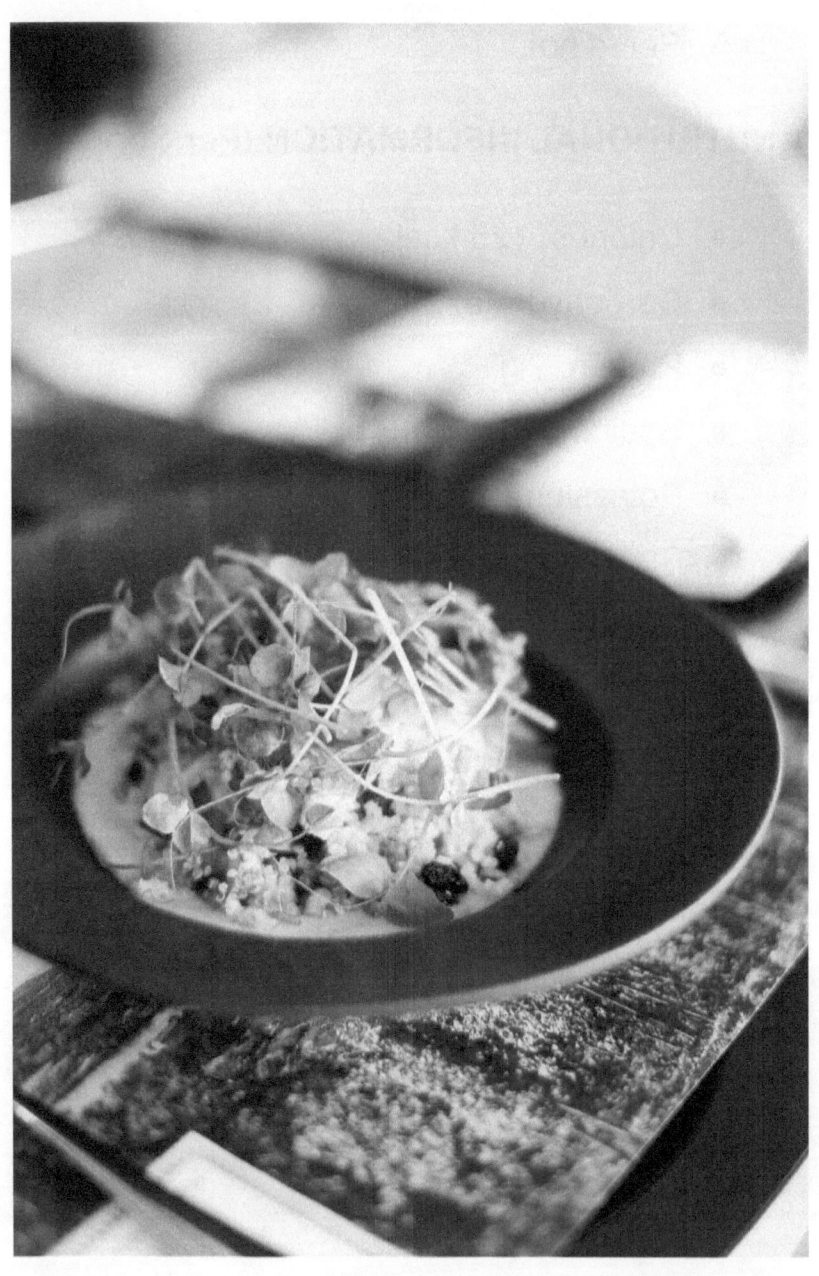

Creamy Crab Soup

COOKING TIME: 15-20 MIN

DESCRIPTION

An awesome soup recipe just like its name denotes - creamy and crabby. This recipe is close to the traditional Maryland eastern shore recipe but with lower potassium ingredients. Great as a family dinner for everyone.

INGREDIENTS FOR 7-8 SERVINGS

- 1 tbsp low salt butter
- 1 cup of white onion, chopped
- ½ pound of fresh crab meat
- 4 cups low salt chicken broth
- 1 cup of soy or vegetable cream
- 2 tbsp cornstarch
- ⅛ tsp dill
- Kosher pepper

METHOD

1. Melt the butter in a large pan over medium heat.
2. Add the onion to the pot and saute until transparent, for around 3 minutes.
3. Add the crab meat to the mix and cook for another couple of minutes.
4. Add the chicken broth to the pan mix and bring to a boil.
5. Mix the vegetable or soy cream with the cornstarch and whisk to combine well. Add to the soup and increase the heat to medium-high.
6. Add the dill and pepper and stir frequently until the soup comes to a boil.
7. Serve hot.

NUTRITIONAL INFORMATION (Per Serving)

- Calories: 89 kcal
- Carbohydrate: 10 g
- Protein: 7 g
- Sodium: 228 mg
- Potassium: 237 mg

- Phosphorus: 83 mg
- Dietary Fiber: 0.3 g
- Fat: 3.7 g
- Sugar: 4.23 g

Broccoli Onion Latkes

COOKING TIME: 10 MIN

DESCRIPTION

A tasty Jewish "latke" recipe with broccoli and onions that you can make in under 10 minutes.

INGREDIENTS FOR 4 SERVINGS

- 3 cups of broccoli florets, roughly chopped
- ½ cup of onion, thinly chopped
- 2 egg whites
- 2 tbsp of all-purpose flour
- 1 tsp of garlic salt
- 2 tbsp of olive oil

METHOD

1. Boil the broccoli in a pot covered with vegetable stock for 5 minutes or until tender.

2. Drain the broccoli and keep it aside. Whisk eggs in a separate bowl and add the flour stirring well.
3. Add the onion into the flour and egg mixture. Add the drained broccoli and combine well.
4. Heat the olive oil in a shallow pan. Drop the mixture with a spoon and flatten with a spatula to make a patty.
5. Shallow fry until golden brown (2 minutes on each side) over medium heat.
6. Place on a dish with absorbing paper and serve hot.

NUTRITIONAL INFORMATION (Per Serving)

- Calories: 110 kcal
- Carbohydrate: 7.2 g
- Protein: 2.9 g
- Sodium: 204 mg
- Potassium: 162 mg
- Phosphorus: 46 mg
- Dietary Fiber: 1.96 g

- Fat: 7 g
- Sugar: 2.5 g

Glazed Carrots

COOKING TIME: 25 MIN

DESCRIPTION

An easy recipe with carrots that you can make as a quick dinner or as a low potassium side dish for rice or meat. Great if you are a vegan as well.

INGREDIENTS FOR 4 SERVINGS

- 2 cups of carrots, sliced into 1" slices
- 1 tbsp of white sugar
- 1 tsp of cornstarch
- 2 tbsp of margarine or vegetable shortening, melted
- ⅛ tsp of salt
- ¼ tsp of ground ginger
- ¼ cup of apple juice

METHOD

1. Poach the carrots in a pan filled with a ¼ cup of boiling water. Cook covered over medium heat until tender (around 12-15 minutes).
2. Combine the sugar, corn starch, ginger, and salt. Add the melted margarine and apple juice and whisk well. Pour the mixture over the carrots in the pan with the water.
3. Allow cooking for around 8-10 minutes or until sauce thickens.

NUTRITIONAL INFORMATION (Per Serving)

- Calories: 101 kcal
- Carbohydrate: 14 g
- Protein: 1 g
- Sodium: 378 g
- Potassium: 202 mg
- Phosphorus: 22.7 mg
- Dietary Fiber: 2.7 g
- Fat: 5 g
- Sugar: 12 g

Slow Cooker Chicken

COOKING TIME: 8 HOURS

DESCRIPTION

If you wish to have some chicken for a family, dinner this slow cooker recipe with just 5 ingredients is all you need. You can also use any leftovers for sandwiches or salads later.

INGREDIENTS FOR 8-9 SERVINGS

- 4 oz. of a whole chicken (uncut)
- 1 tbsp of all-purpose or chicken seasoning
- ½ tsp of black pepper
- ½ tsp of garlic powder
- 3 tbsp of wine

METHOD

1. Wash the chicken and remove any insides.

2. Wrap with the chicken seasoning, garlic powder, and pepper.
3. Place in a lightly greased slow cooker/crock-pot, add the wine and cover with the lid and set to low heat for 8 hours.
4. Remove the skin, cut, and serve.

NUTRITIONAL INFORMATION (Per Serving)

- Calories: 131 kcal
- Carbohydrate: 0 g
- Protein: 7 g
- Sodium: 60 mg
- Potassium: 160 mg
- Phosphorus: 130 mg
- Dietary Fiber: 0 g
- Fat: 6 g
- Sugar: 0.25 g

Syrian Style Lamb Kafta

COOKING TIME: 18-20 MIN

DESCRIPTION

Kafta is a traditional middle eastern lamb dish that is best made on the charcoal grill, however, you can also make this in the oven's grill for convenience reasons. Serve ideally with chopped cucumber and tomatoes.

INGREDIENTS FOR 6 SERVINGS

- 1 pound of finely ground lamb
- 1 tsp of cumin
- 1 tsp of paprika
- 1 tsp of sumac or lemon pepper
- 2 cloves of garlic, minced
- 3 tbsp of chopped parsley
- 1 tbsp of olive oil
- ½ tsp of salt

METHOD

1. Combine all the ingredients and mix well with your hands.
2. Preheat your oven's broiler.
3. Take 6 medium wooden sticks (for skewers) and wrap each with approx. 2 inches of the mixture.
4. Cook over a baking sheet for approx. 8-10 minutes on each side.

NUTRITIONAL INFORMATION (Per Serving)

- Calories: 170 kcal
- Carbohydrate: 0.8 g
- Protein: 13.5 g
- Sodium: 45 mg
- Potassium: 215 mg
- Phosphorus: 147 mg
- Dietary Fiber: 0.5 g
- Fat: 11.7 g
- Sugar: 0 g

Spicy Lime Shrimp

COOKING TIME: 5 MIN

DESCRIPTION

A spicy and tangy shrimp recipe inspired by the Creole seafood flavors of New Orleans. If you are a fan of peppers and lime, you'll love this one.

INGREDIENTS FOR 4-5 SERVINGS

- 32 large shrimp, peeled and deveined
- ¼ cup of lime juice
- 1 garlic clove, minced
- 1 green onion, sliced
- 3 tbsp of red bell pepper, diced
- 2 tbsp of fresh cilantro, chopped
- 1 tsp of jalapeno chili, minced
- ⅛ tsp of salt
- 1 big cucumber, sliced

METHOD

1. To make your dressing, combine the lime juice, green onion, jalapeno chili, cilantro, garlic, and oil or salt in a mixing bowl.
2. In a separate mixing bowl, add the shrimps with 3 tbsp of the lime juice marinade. Cover and let in the fridge for 40 minutes.
3. Turn on your oven's broiler. Discard the shrimp from the lime marinade and broil for around 3-4 minutes in total or 2 minutes on each side.
4. Take off the heat and pour the remaining marinade on top.
5. Place over the cucumber slices and serve cold.

NUTRITIONAL INFORMATION (Per Serving)

- Calories: 132 kcal
- Carbohydrate: 3 g
- Protein: 12 g
- Sodium: 149 mg
- Potassium: 202 mg

- Phosphorus: 128 mg
- Dietary Fiber: 0.6 g
- Fat: 8 g
- Sugar: 1.4 g

Pasta Shells with Peas and Bacon

COOKING TIME: 12 MIN

DESCRIPTION

If you are a fan of comfort and rich flavors, this pasta dish with bacon, cream and peas will definitely become a favorite. The addition of parmesan cheese and butter makes it extra fragrant, without increasing its potassium levels.

INGREDIENTS FOR 6 SERVINGS

- 1 cup of whole wheat pasta shells (you may also use penne pasta)
- ¾ cup of frozen peas
- 2 tbsp of unsalted butter
- ½ cup of parmesan cheese, grated
- 3 slices of bacon,
- 1 cup of white onion, chopped
- 2-3 cloves of garlic, minced

- ¼ tsp of kosher pepper
- 1 tbsp of lemon juice

METHOD

1. Boil the pasta into a pot filled with 1 liter of boiling water for 8-10 minutes (or according to packaging instructions). Add the peas during the last two minutes of cooking. Drain and keep the water aside.
2. Cut the butter with a knife into small chunks. Combine the ricotta and parmesan cheese in a separate big bowl to mix with pasta later.
3. Cut the bacon into thin strips and heat a skillet with cooking spray. Shallow fry until nice and crisp but not burned (around 6 minutes). Remove and set aside.

4. Add the onion to the same pan and cook until transparent, for approx. 3 minutes.
5. Add the minced garlic and saute for another minute. Transfer the onion and bacon mixture to a cheese bowl.
6. Add ½ cup of the cooking water kept and the lemon juice to the cheese mixture. Add the drained pasta with the peas and toss to coat evenly.
7. Finish with the cooked bacon strips and some pepper to taste.
8. Serve warm.

NUTRITIONAL INFORMATION (Per Serving)

- Calories: 313 kcal
- Carbohydrate: 27 g
- Protein: 13 g
- Sodium: 244 g
- Potassium: 172 mg
- Phosphorus: 203 mg
- Dietary Fiber: 3.3 g

- Fat: 14 g
- Sugar: 2.6 g

Buffalo Chicken Wings

COOKING TIME: 35 MIN

DESCRIPTION

An all-American dish, buffalo chicken wings are a famous dinner and side dish in football and festive nights. And the best part is that each counts only 105 mg of potassium per serving so feel free to eat as much as 5 wings.

INGREDIENTS FOR 12 SERVINGS

- 24 chicken wings (drumettes)
- ¼ cup of low sodium tomato sauce
- 8 tbsp of unsalted butter,
- ⅓ cup of hot pepper sauce e.g. Tabasco
- ½ tsp of garlic
- 1 tbsp of olive oil
- ½ tsp of Italian seasoning mix
- ¼ cup roasted red bell pepper puree/sauce.

METHOD

1. Preheat your oven 400F/190C.
2. Melt your butter in a pan.
3. Pour in the hot pepper sauce, tomato sauce, garlic powder, olive oil, and Italian seasoning. Mix well with a spatula. Let heat for 2 minutes and remove from the heat.
4. Arrange the chicken wings on a baking sheet.
5. Brush the sauce over the chicken wings, making sure they are evenly coated, and bake for 30-35 minutes.

NUTRITIONAL INFORMATION (Per Serving)

- Calories: 131 kcal
- Carbohydrate: 0.1 g
- Protein: 8 g
- Sodium: 64 mg
- Potassium: 105 mg
- Phosphorus: 61 mg
- Dietary Fiber: 0 g
- Fat: 11 g

- Sugar: 0.5 g

Cauliflower and Apple Soup

COOKING TIME: 40 MIN

DESCRIPTION

A delicious vegetarian soup that blends ideally the flavors of cauliflower and apples with herbs and bread crostini as an optional addition on top. Perfect for family weekend dinner.

INGREDIENTS FOR 12 SERVINGS

- 1 head of cauliflower, chopped into small chunks
- 1 cup of white onion, diced
- 1 cup of apple, thinly cubed
- 2 cloves of garlic, minced
- 6 cups of chicken stock
- 1 tsp of thyme,
- 1 tsp of rosemary
- 1 tsp of sage
- 12 baguette slices
- 1 tbsp of garlic powder

METHOD

1. To make the bread and garlic crostini, drizzle the baguette slices with olive oil, minced garlic, and garlic powder. Bake in a preheated oven at 350F/175C for 10 minutes. Keep aside.
2. To make the soup, bring the chicken stock to a boil and add the vegetables, the apple, and the rest ingredients. Let cook with the lid covered for 25-30 minutes.
3. Transfer the soup to a deep soup dish and blend with a hand immersion blender.
4. Serve in individual soup bowls with some sliced bread crostini on top.

NUTRITIONAL INFORMATION (Per Serving)

- Calories: 82 kcal
- Carbohydrate: 15 g
- Protein: 3 g
- Sodium: 125 mg

- Potassium: 231 mg
- Phosphorus: 64 mg
- Dietary Fiber: 2 g
- Fat: 1.1 g
- Sugar: 2.63 g

Mapo's Tofu and Pork

COOKING TIME: 15 MIN

DESCRIPTION

A traditional Chinese dish with tofu and pork as the main ingredients with a spicy and slightly oily sauce. You can make it with shrimps or chicken in place of the pork if you wish.

INGREDIENTS FOR 8 SERVINGS

- 3 oz/120 gr of ground pork
- 1 block (350gr) medium-firm tofu
- 2 cloves of garlic, minced
- 1 tsp of red chili flakes
- 1 green onion, sliced

For the marinade

- 1 tbsp of sesame oil
- 1 tsp of low sodium soy sauce
- 1 tsp rice vinegar or dry white wine
- 1 tbsp of vegetable oil

- ½ tsp of white sugar

For the sauce

- 1/s tsp low sodium sauce
- 1 tsp of sesame oil
- 3 tbsp of water
- 1 tbsp of cornstarch

METHOD

1. Mix all the marinade ingredients in a bowl. Add the pork and allow to marinate for approx. 15 minutes.
2. Mix all the sauce ingredients in a separate bowl and keep aside.
3. Heat the vegetable oil in a wok or skillet and saute the garlic with the chili flakes. Add the pork and stir-fry until fully cooked and no longer pink.
4. Add the tofu and stir gently to mix with the rest of the ingredients.
5. Stir in the sauce mix and stir repeatedly until it thickens.

6. Garnish optionally with a few spring onion slices.
7. Serve warm.

NUTRITIONAL INFORMATION (Per Serving)

- Calories: 110 kcal
- Carbohydrate: 3.3 g
- Protein: 7.4 g
- Sodium: 35 mg
- Potassium: 102 mg
- Phosphorus: 68 mg
- Dietary Fiber: 0.7 g
- Fat: 8.5 g
- Sugar: 0.2 g

Lemon Orzo Salad

COOKING TIME: 10 MIN

DESCRIPTION

A lovely pasta salad with lemon, orzo, and other herbs that is perfect for spring or summer evenings with friends or family. Great as next day much at work too.

INGREDIENTS FOR 4 SERVINGS

- 1 cup of orzo pasta
- 1 tsp of chicken bouillon granules
- 1 green onion, diced
- 1 red bell pepper, diced
- 2 tbsp of tarragon, chopped
- 2 tbsp of fresh parsley leaves, chopped
- 1 clove of garlic, minced
- 2 tbsp of lemon juice
- 1 tbsp of olive oil

METHOD

1. Cook the orzo in 3 cups of boiling water with the bouillon granules dissolved for 10-12 minutes (or based on package instructions).
2. Rinse with cold water and drain. Keep aside.
3. Add the rest of the ingredients to a salad bowl, toss to combine well, and serve cool.

NUTRITIONAL INFORMATION (Per Serving)

- Calories: 148 kcal
- Carbohydrate: 24 g
- Protein: 4 g
- Sodium: 7 mg
- Potassium: 164 mg
- Phosphorus: 65 mg
- Dietary Fiber: 1.6 g
- Fat: 4 g
- Sugar: 1.4 g

Sausage Stuffed Jalapenos

COOKING TIME: 20 MIN

DESCRIPTION

Delicious dinner recipe with ground pork sausage, cheese, and spices as the filling for roasted jalapeno boats.

INGREDIENTS FOR 12 SERVINGS.

- 1 pound of ground pork sausage
- 1 oz. of low fat and softened cream cheese
- 1 cup of ranch dressing (optional)
- 1 cup of parmesan cheese, grated

METHOD

1. Preheat the oven at 400F/190C.
2. Place the ground sausage in a skillet over medium heat and cook until brown. Drain and set aside.

3. Combine the sausage, cream cheese, and parmesan cheese in a mixing bowl.
4. Fill the jalapeno halves with approx. 1 tbsp of the mixture each.
5. Place over a baking sheet and bake in the oven for 20 minutes.

NUTRITIONAL INFORMATION (Per Serving)

- Calories: 362 kcal
- Carbohydrate: 4.3 g
- Protein: 9.2 g
- Sodium: 601 mg
- Potassium: 199 mg
- Phosphorus: 68 mg
- Dietary Fiber: 1.1 g
- Fat: 34.2 g
- Sugar: 0.16 g

Desserts

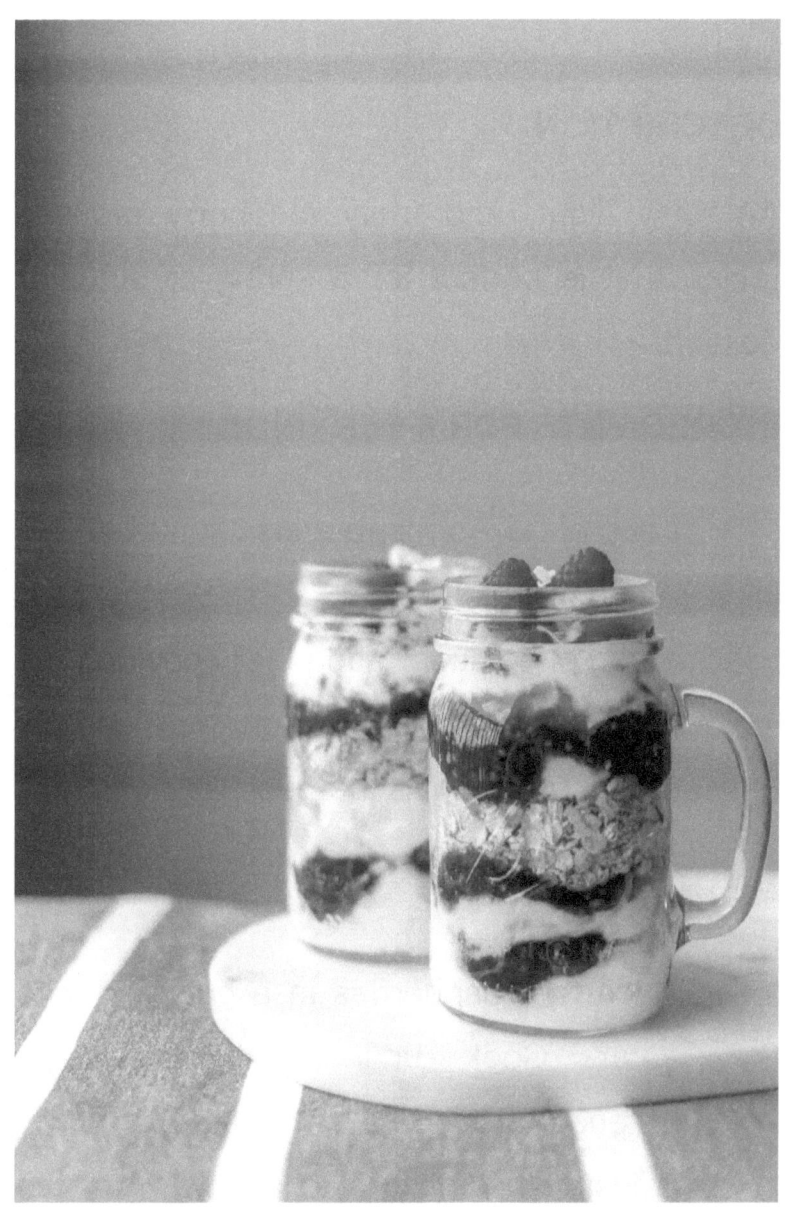

Raspberry Mousse

COOKING TIME: 12 MIN

DESCRIPTION

An easy, light, and fruity raspberry mousse recipe that is perfect for a spring or summer dessert.

INGREDIENTS FOR 6 SERVINGS.

- 1 cup of frozen raspberries
- ¼ cup of water
- 2 tbsp of no sugar added jelly powder
- 1 ½ cup of whipping cream
- 1 pack of fresh raspberries

METHOD

1. Place the raspberries in a pot filled with water. Cook until raspberries have softened (around 10-12 minutes).
2. Transfer the mixture to a bowl. Add the jelly powder and stir well to dissolve.

3. Once the mixture has cooled down, add in the whipping cream. Distribute the mixture into 6 dessert bowls or glasses.
4. Chill for at least a couple of hours before serving.
5. Garnish with a tbsp of fresh raspberries on top of each serving.

NUTRITIONAL INFORMATION (Per Serving)

- Calories: 94 kcal
- Carbohydrate: 20.1 g
- Protein: 1.1 g
- Sodium: 22 mg
- Potassium: 133 mg
- Phosphorus: 28 mg
- Dietary Fiber: 5.2 g
- Fat: 1.61 g
- Sugar: 1.8 g

Honey Ginger Cookies

COOKING TIME: 10 MIN

DESCRIPTION

A lovely cookie recipe with ginger if you wish to bake something fast and enjoy it with your afternoon coffee or tea. You can also keep these up to two weeks.

INGREDIENTS FOR 15 SERVINGS

(30 cookies)

- 2 cups of all-purpose flour
- ¾ cups of vegetable shortening
- 1 cup of white sugar
- ¼ cup honey
- 2 tsp of baking soda
- 1 tsp of ginger powder
- 1 ¼ tsp of cinnamon
- 1 tsp of ground cloves
- A bit of icing sugar (for the top)

METHOD

1. Preheat the oven to 325 F/175C.
2. Combine all the cream/wet ingredients in a mixing bowl and beat well.
3. In a separate bowl, sift the flour and combine it with the sugar and all the other ingredients.
4. Add the wet ingredients into the dry mixture and mix fast and well.
5. Roll into balls with your hands and place over a greased paper sheet, making sure each cookie ball is at least 1 inch apart from the other.
6. Bake for 8-10 minutes.

NUTRITIONAL INFORMATION (Per Serving)

- Calories: 112 kcal
- Carbohydrate: 16 g
- Protein: 1 g
- Sodium: 90 mg
- Potassium: 18 mg
- Phosphorus: 13 mg
- Dietary Fiber: 0.4 g

- Fat: 5 g
- Sugar: 17.9 g

Honey Baked Pear

COOKING TIME: 30 MIN

DESCRIPTION

A nice alternative version to the classic poached pear recipe, baked in the oven and enhanced with 5 spices for extra aroma and flavor.

INGREDIENTS FOR 8 SERVINGS

- 4 pears, peeled and halved
- ¼ cup of unsalted butter or margarine
- ¼ cup of lemon juice
- ½ tsp of 5-spice powder
- 1 tsp of orange zest
- 1 tsp of vanilla extract

METHOD

1. Preheat the oven at 350F/175C.
2. Pour the lemon juice over the pears to avoid any darkening.

3. Mix the melted butter, spices, zest, and vanilla in a bowl. Pour over the pears.
4. Place the marinated pears in an oven-safe pan and bake for 25-30 minutes.
5. Serve warm.

NUTRITIONAL INFORMATION (Per Serving)

- Calories: 141 kcal
- Carbohydrate: 23 g
- Protein: 0.5 g
- Sodium: 2 mg
- Potassium: 121 mg
- Phosphorus: 12 mg
- Dietary Fiber: 2.7 g
- Fat: 6 g
- Sugar: 8.4 g

Watermelon Sorbet

COOKING TIME: 1 MIN

DESCRIPTION

Refreshing and cooling sorbet recipe that is perfect for chilling during hot summer days (and nights). It has only 52 calories per serving so no need to worry about ruining your weight loss diet.

INGREDIENTS FOR 2 SERVINGS

- 1 cup of ice, crushed
- 1 cup of watermelon chunks, seeded
- 2 tbsp of lime juice
- 1 tbsp of sugar
- 2 small watermelon slices (for garnishing)

METHOD

1. Pulse all the ingredients except for the watermelon slices in a blender for 30 seconds to 1 minute.

2. Pour the mixture into 2 mason jars or glasses, top with the wedges, and serve chilled immediately.

NUTRITIONAL INFORMATION (Per Serving)

- Calories: 52 kcal
- Carbohydrate: 13 g
- Protein: 0 g
- Sodium: 1 mg
- Potassium: 96 mg
- Phosphorus: 9 mg
- Dietary Fiber: 0.3 g
- Fat: 0 g
- Sugar: 107.2 g

Aunt Tula's Carrot Cake

COOKING TIME: 50 MIN

DESCRIPTION

A recipe close to the traditional old school carrot cake recipe with a bit of a twist. Make it and serve with your daily coffee or tea. Good for ladies' parties as well.

INGREDIENTS FOR 20 SERVINGS.

- 2 cups all-purpose flour
- 1 cup of white sugar
- 3 cups of carrot
- 1 cup of vegetable oil
- 4 large eggs, beaten
- 2 tbsp of skimmed milk
- 8 oz. of cream cheese
- ¼ cup unsalted butter
- 2 tsp of cinnamon
- 1 tsp of vanilla extract
- 2 tsp vanilla powder

- 1 cup of icing sugar

METHOD

1. Preheat the oven at 350F/180C.
2. In a large mixing bowl, combine all the dry ingredients e.g. flour, sugar, and others. Slowly incorporate the oil, the beaten eggs, the vanilla, and the milk. Mix well until the mixture is uniform and slightly fluffy.
3. Pour the cake batter onto a lightly greased cake pan (around 9x11 inches)
4. Bake for 45-50 minutes
5. In a separate mixing bowl, beat the cream cheese with the icing sugar and vanilla powder to make your frosting.
6. Spread over the cooled carrot cake with a flat spatula. Slice and serve.

NUTRITIONAL INFORMATION (Per Serving)

- Calories: 324 kcal
- Carbohydrate: 34 g

- Protein: 4 g
- Sodium: 180.7 mg
- Potassium: 98 mg
- Phosphorus: 54 mg
- Dietary Fiber: 1 g
- Fat: 19 g
- Sugar: 23.34 g

Conclusion

As specified earlier, while we have made an effort to include in this Renal Diet Cookbook recipes that are low in potassium, sodium, and phosphorus, it's best to consult with your doctor or nutritionist when trying out new recipes to confirm that the amounts and limits of the above key nutrients are suitable for your renal damage stage. Those that are currently on an earlier stage of CKD, for example, may consume up to 2000 mg of potassium per day, throughout their daily meals, which is a relatively easy target, considering that the average person consumes around 2500 mg of potassium or less per day. Respectively, the total daily intake of phosphorus should not surpass 600 mg (per day) but since most recipes contain less than 150 mg of phosphorus, this target isn't hard to achieve. Finally, the daily limit of sodium for renal patients with potential diabetes and/or heart disease should be up to 1500 mg/day.

If you know exactly the nutritional info for each recipe, as in the case of this book, it's also recommended to keep a journal of the meals/recipes you consume per day and show it to your doctor so you can both track your diet habits better.

Please always consult with your family doctor or nutritionist before using a current recipe or the diet program.

Thanks for your attention!

Written by: Albert Simon
Copyright © 2021.
All rights reserved.

All Rights Reserved. No part of this publication or the information in it may be quoted from or reproduced in any form by means such as printing, scanning, photocopying, or otherwise without prior written permission of the copyright holder.

Disclaimer and Terms of Use: Effort has been made to ensure that the information in this book is accurate and complete, however, the author and the publisher do not warrant the accuracy of the information, text, and graphics contained within the book due to the rapidly changing nature of science, research, known and unknown facts, and internet. The Author and the publisher do not hold any responsibility for errors, omissions, or contrary interpretation of the subject matter herein. This book is presented solely for motivational and informational purposes only.

www.ingramcontent.com/pod-product-compliance
Lightning Source LLC
Chambersburg PA
CBHW020631220526
45464CB00001B/108